PRINCIPLES OF BIOMEDICAL ENGINEERING FOR NURSING STAFF

PRINCIPLES OF BIOMEDICAL ENGINEERING FOR NURSING STAFF

HANS A. VON DER MOSEL

OXFORD

BLACKWELL SCIENTIFIC PUBLICATIONS

LONDON EDINBURGH BOSTON

MELBOURNE PARIS BERLIN VIENNA

R856
.M65513
1994

Contents

Preface

New medical technology has become increasingly complex over the last 40 years. Many medical and nursing schools have failed to keep pace with this development and to introduce lectures and practical courses to promote the understanding of high-tech medical care. It is therefore not surprising that these new machines, created to save human life, in some cases become a source of accidents. Most of these accidents are caused not by technical failure, but by incorrect and sometimes even careless handling by their users who are simply overwhelmed by the new technology for which they were not prepared during their education and training.

This book aims to help those who have to work with electromedical equipment on a daily basis to gain a better understanding of the underlying functional principles of such equipment and also to learn about the possible hazards involved in its applications. It has been written primarily for nursing staff. In order to publish it at a reasonable price that a nurse can afford, it cannot be a comprehensive manual of all of the equipment available on the market. The equipment selected is commonly found in hospital wards, special units and most doctors' surgeries. The author has made a great effort to present the material in such a way that it can be understood without a detailed knowledge of engineering sciences, physics and mathematics. It is hoped that the book will contribute towards a better understanding of such equipment and towards a reduction in the number of accidents caused by users.

The author wishes to thank all of those who have given him valuable help by contributing suggestions, critical comments and information as well as by supplying illustrative material. There are just too many of them to name personally.

However, the author wishes to express his gratitude to Mrs Lisa Field, Mrs Caroline Savage and Mrs Mary Sayers as well as to all staff of Blackwell Scientific Publications for their friendly cooperation and for much good advice during the production of the book, and to Ms Rosemary Webster who, as a reviewer for the publisher, made valuable suggestions about improvements. The author also owes special thanks to Mrs Helga Juckel, Chief Editor of the German nursing journal *Die Schwester – Der Pfleger*, who had the idea for such a book, and, last but not least, to his wife Christine who helped considerably with her patience and her critical review of the manuscript.

Any suggestions for improvement or expansion for later editions of this book are always very welcome.

Professor Hans A. von der Mosel
Augsburg, Germany, July 1993

Part I
Introduction

Chapter 1
An Introduction to Electricity

The electrical accident – causes and prevention

For most of us electricity is an important part of our daily life, so much so in fact that the possible dangers connected with its use are not appreciated by most people.

If we look at the subject of electricity in medicine, it must be acknowledged that accidents caused by the use of electricity are not as rare as we would like to believe. Most such accidents are caused not by faulty equipment but rather by mistakes made by the users of such equipment. By 1972 the author had published a statistical evaluation of the causes of about 1600 serious accidents with electromedical apparatus which were, to a large degree, investigated by himself. It was concluded that about 64% of these accidents were clearly caused by user errors or careless handling of equipment. At the time these results triggered vehement criticism. However, verification of these findings was soon obtained. In 1986 the government of the then Federal Republic of Germany introduced medical device safety legislation and made mandatory the reporting of accidents and near-accidents. Since then, 68 serious accidents have been reported of which 67 were unquestionably caused by user error.

Expensive life-saving or life-supporting equipment loses its usefulness if patients are subsequently injured or even killed through its use. For many years, and so far without success, the author has tried to convince the authorities to introduce mandatory lectures and examinations on medical equipment technology into the curricula of medical and nursing schools. It is not acceptable that physicians and nurses should be constantly at risk of facing legal consequences because of incorrect handling of technical equipment just because their training does not provide them with the necessary knowledge.

In order to avoid accidents with technical equipment, knowledge of some simple basic rules of the physics of electricity as well as a solid knowledge of the equipment, its correct handling and the dangers involved, is absolutely necessary.

How much electricity is dangerous for human beings?

The usual answer in reply to this question ranges from about 50 to 1 000 volts. This illustrates just how ignorant most people are about the concept of electricity. Electric current must flow in order for electricity to be dangerous, and electric current is in fact measured in amperes (or amps for short), not in volts.

In an electrical system there are three important units of measurement, the volt, the ohm and the ampere. These measure the potential difference, the resistance and the electric current respectively. It is easier to understand the invisible medium of electricity if we draw an analogy with a visible medium such as water. Let us consider a water supply system where three similar components can be seen: the water pressure, the resistance and the rate of flow of water per unit of time.

The force at which the water moves around the system is the water pressure. It corresponds, when transferred to the electrical system, to what is known as the voltage, also called the potential difference or electromagnetic force (emf), i.e. the unit of electrical pressure, which is determined by the electrical generator and measured in volts.

The resistance within the water supply system is determined primarily by the amount the tap is opened. Resistance is greatest when the tap is closed. Within the electrical system this corresponds to the resistance in ohms which is caused mainly by fixed or adjustable electrical and electronic components within the equipment.

The rate of flow of water in a given amount of time at the tap is the result of the water pressure and the resistance. The more the tap is turned on, the lower is the resistance, and the greater the flow of water in any given time. Within the electrical system, the amount of electricity flowing within a given amount of time will be the electrical current measured in amperes. The higher the resistance (in ohms), the lower the flow of electrical current (in amperes).

The danger of electrical currents

The interaction between electrical current, voltage and resistance was discovered by the German physicist Georg Simon Ohm (1787–1854). Ohm's law states, in short, that if you know two electrical values, you can calculate the third one using this law. The law is expressed mathematically as:

volts   = amperes × resistance
amperes   = volts ÷ resistance
resistance = volts ÷ amperes

There is an even more simple way to find the correct formula for calculating Ohm's law:

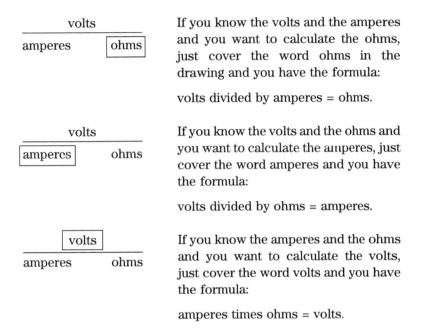

If you know the volts and the amperes and you want to calculate the ohms, just cover the word ohms in the drawing and you have the formula:

volts divided by amperes = ohms.

If you know the volts and the ohms and you want to calculate the amperes, just cover the word amperes and you have the formula:

volts divided by ohms = amperes.

If you know the amperes and the ohms and you want to calculate the volts, just cover the word volts and you have the formula:

amperes times ohms = volts.

You will probably never have to make these calculations, but it is useful to know how simple such calculations are.

However, before we can answer the question asked at the beginning of this chapter, i.e. how much electricity is dangerous for human beings?, we need to consider other factors.

Three factors are important when considering the seriousness of an electrical accident and the danger of electricity:

(1) The *amount of current* which will flow through the victim in the event of an electrical accident.
(2) The *electrical pathway*, i.e. the way electricity will pass through the body of the victim.
(3) The *current density*, which will be discussed later in this chapter.

The amount of current, or current quantity, is the amount of electrical current as described previously, expressed in amperes.

The electrical pathway, or current pathway, is a very important factor which determines the hazard. If, for example, the current enters through one finger of a hand and flows out through another finger of the same hand, it may cause severe burns on this hand along the current pathway, but the victim's life is at no time in danger.

If, however, the current enters through one hand and leaves through another extremity, for example from one hand to the other hand, vital organs such as the heart, the lungs, the spinal cord etc. are within the current pathway and could be influenced or even damaged in such a way that the victim's life is endangered.

How the body reacts to various levels of electrical current

Kouwenhoven and Milnor (1957) and Dalziel (1959) independently investigated the effects of electrical current on the human body and drew the same conclusions. They considered the effects of different amounts of an alternating current (AC) of 50–60 Hz on a body where the current pathway was from one extremity to another. Their results were as follows.

1 milliampere (1 mA = 0.001 amperes)

This is the amount of current which can just be felt by intact skin as a slight tingling sensation. On damaged skin (wounds, etc.) or at mucous membranes, about half this amount of current can be detected.

16 milliamperes (16 mA = 0.016 amperes)

If a person grasps, with their hand, an electrical conductor which carries this amount of current, the victim will not be able to remove their hand from the conductor. The flexor muscles of the hand are stimulated considerably more than the extensors, and the hand 'grasps'. However, there is no immediate danger to life.

As the amount of current increases, the delivered current will become increasingly painful. The very strong muscular contractions lead to mechanical damage of muscles and/or bones. However, despite severe pain and exhaustion, the functioning of the heart and lungs is not greatly affected.

50 milliamperes (50 mA = 0.05 amperes)

Death may occur by suffocation, since with such electrical stimulation the chest and respiratory muscles will contract spasmodically, preventing the victim from breathing normally.

100 milliamperes (100 mA = 0.1 amperes)

If the amount of current increases still further, to about 100 mA, cardiac fibrillation will occur. If the current is not stopped immediately and defibrillation initiated, this will cause death of the victim in a very short time. With these levels of current passing across the human body, severe internal burn injuries as well as irreversible respiratory paralysis and/or cerebral hypoxia are almost always the usual result.

3 amperes or greater

At currents of more than 3 amperes (3 A), the cardiac muscle contracts as a result of the very strong stimulation and remains in this position. The heart no longer pumps, the circulation collapses, and the victim dies.

For the sake of completeness it should be mentioned here that very short pulses of electrical current of about this strength are used for cardiac defibrillation. The current is applied directly to the heart and does not influence the chest and respiratory muscles. Subsequently, the heart remains, for a short period of time, in the contracted position and ideally begins to beat normally again thereafter.

The above results occur when an electrical current is applied through normal, intact skin. However, if the electrical current is applied by bypassing the skin, i.e. invasively, the situation is quite different. To draw another analogy the human body may be represented by a leather bag filled with a saline solution. Whereas the leather has a relatively high resistance to electricity, saline solutions are good electrical conductors. Hence, in this case it needs only a very small electrical current to produce serious damage.

According to the investigations of Whalen, Starmer and McIntosh (1964), only about 250 microamperes (250 μA = 0.250 milliamperes = 0.000 250 amperes), depending on the current density, may be sufficient to produce cardiac fibrillation caused by the electricity being conducted via the circulatory system directly to the heart. In several cases this was found to occur at only 20 microamperes (20 μA = 0.020 milliamperes = 0.000 020 amperes).

How can such currents get into the human body?

As we now know, the ampere is the unit of measurement obtained by dividing the volt by the ohm. Regarding the current pathway through the human body, the resistance opposing the current is primarily caused by the skin. Normal human skin has a resistance of about 1000 ohms per cm^2. However, quite large differences are possible regarding this resistance. Callous skin on hands and feet may, in the case of dry skin, have a resistance of up to 1 million ohms. In the case of moist skin, however, the normal skin resistance may be as low as 500 ohms or less.

Let us first look at a skin having a resistance of 1000 ohms per cm^2. If a person having such a skin resistance comes into contact with 220 volts AC, i.e. with the normal European power supply voltage (in the USA it is 110 volts AC), the resulting amount of current would be $220 \div 1000 = 0.22$ amperes, or 220 milliamperes (in the USA it would be $110 \div 1000 = 0.11$ amperes or 110 milliamperes). As we now know, this is sufficient to cause cardiac fibrillation and severe internal burns as well as irreversible respiratory paralysis and/or cerebral hypoxia.

In the case of severely ill people in an intensive care unit, the situation is even more dangerous. If the patient has a fever and is sweating, the skin resistance may be reduced to 250 ohms. If the patient is connected to an ECG monitor, the contact gel at the electrodes may cause a further reduction of the skin resistance to about 100 ohms. Using the same calculation as above, $220 \div 100 = 2.2$ amperes (in the USA $110 \div 100 = 1.1$ amperes) can flow through the patient!

Instead of the power supply voltage of 220 (110) volts, if we now look at the 'low safety voltage' of 25 volts as found in most electromedical apparatus, then $25 \div 100 = 0.25$ amperes (250 milliamperes) would flow through the patient with the results already described.

If, however, electricity can enter the human body by circumventing the skin resistance barrier, for example through an infusion cannula or through the electrode of an external cardiac pacemaker, the resistance opposing such current would be a maximum of 10 ohms. If we now apply the already mentioned 'low safety voltage' of 25 volts, there will in this case be a current of $25 \div 10 = 2.5$ amperes, an extremely dangerous level that will cause cardiac fibrillation and severe internal burns as well as, depending upon the current pathway, irreversible respiratory paralysis and/or cerebral hypoxia. Therefore, extreme care is needed with patients where blood pressure is measured invasively or who are connected to an external cardiac pacemaker or similar equipment. The current density already mentioned will also be of importance. If current reaches the patient through a larger conductive area (e.g. an infusion

needle, where not only the tip, but the entire metallic surface is conductive), we have a so-called low current density and the current, on
entering the patient, will be distributed over the entire conductive area
which is not quite as dangerous. However, if electrical current is applied
through a very small conductive area, e.g. the tip of a cardiac pacemaker
electrode, the current density is high and the hazard is accordingly more
serious.

In order to explain the term 'current density' even more clearly, the
example of 'electrical high-frequency surgery' may be used. The active,
i.e. current supplying, electrode has a very small contact area (or high
current density) which enables it to perform its function of cutting or
coagulation. The same amount of current will be carried away from
the patient without doing any harm to the skin at this location by
using the passive electrode which is a large area (low current density)
electrode.

As has already been mentioned, depending on the current pathway an
electrical current of 250 microamperes will be sufficient if applied
invasively to the human body to trigger a cardiac fibrillation. In order to
obtain a current of 250 microamperes, only $0.000\,025 \times 10 = 0.002\,500$
volts ($= 2.5$ millivolts) are necessary. Such a low voltage is present within
all electrical and electronic equipment.

These voltages are derived by induction from magnetic fields which
occur around every current-carrying part of the equipment, and also
from many other sources. They are generally called stray currents. If the
equipment is properly earthed, such stray currents will be carried to
earth and hence will not cause any harm. However, if the earthing
connector is interrupted, they will be present at any electrically conductive part of the equipment.

As we know from the investigations of Kouwenhoven and Milnor
(1957) and of Dalziel (1959), the smallest amount of current we can feel
is around 0.5 to 1 milliampere ($0.000\,5$ to 0.001 ampere). So just under
500 microamperes would not be felt by any healthy, normal person.
Therefore, it is quite possible that if you have your hand on a cardiac
pacemaker electrode connector, the cannula of invasive blood pressure
apparatus or similar, when adjusting equipment, you may conduct this
amount of electrical current along your own body surface to the patient
without your realizing it. The patient, however, gets the full force of this
current and reacts with cardiac fibrillation without your realizing what
has happened.

Conclusion

It should now be clear why extreme care is necessary with all invasive measures concerning your patient, and why it is very important that the equipment should have regular safety inspections. Connector leads linking the equipment to the power supply should be inspected at least every 6 months to ensure that earthing connectors are functioning properly.

Accidents do not just happen out of the blue. In most cases, accidents with this kind of medical equipment are caused by faults within the equipment or by careless and/or ignorant use by the operator. Unavoidable true accidents are quite rare events. Full attention and very careful handling are absolutely vital when using all such equipment.

References

Dalziel, C.F. (1959) The effects of electrical shock in man, US Atomic Energy Commission Safety Technical Bulletin 7.

Kouwenhoven, W.B. and Milnor, W. R. (1957) Field treatment in electric shock cases, *Electrical Engineering* **76.**

Whalen, R.E., Starmer, C.F. and McIntosh, H.D. (1964) Electrical hazards associated with cardiac pacemaking, *Ann. New York Acad. Sci.* **111**, 922.

Further reading

Anonymous (1960) Medicine and the law: fatal shock from a cardiac monitor, *Lancet* **1.**

Bruner, J.M.R. (1967) Hazards of electrical apparatus, *Anesthesiology* **28**, 2.

Gechman, R. (1967) The tiny flaws in medical design can kill, *Electronic Design* **18**.

Lee, W.R. (1964) The nature and management of electric shock', *Brit. J. Anaesth.* **36**.

von der Mosel, H.A. (1968) The electrical microshock hazard, *US Safety News.*

von der Mosel, H.A. (1970) Is your intensive care unit electrically safe?, *Med. Surg. Review.*

von der Mosel, H.A. (1970) ICU and CCU safety, *Med. Electronics & Data* **1**, 6, 76.

von der Mosel, H.A. (1971) Der klinisch-biomedizinische Ingenieur, *Schweiz. Arztezeitg.* **52**, 52.

von der Mosel, H.A. (1990) Umsetzung der Medizingeräteverordnung in privat-ärztlichen Praxen, *MT Medizintechnik* **3**, 105–106.

Nordijk, J.A. *et al.* (1961) Myocardial electrodes and the danger of ventricular fibrillation, *Lancet* **1**.

Stanley, P. (1967) Monitors that save lives can also kill, *The Modern Hospital* **108**, 3.

Chapter 2
Avoiding Accidents with Technical Equipment – Basic Safety Rules

There are a number of basic rules that should be applied when operating technical equipment in order to avoid accidents. The consequences of not taking precautions can be serious injury or can even be fatal.

Rule 1

If equipment is to be disconnected from the power supply, always disconnect the power cord from the wall socket before disconnecting the power cord from the equipment. Conversely, if equipment is to be connected to the power supply, always connect the power cord first to the equipment and thereafter to the socket outlet.

Rule 2

Never use multiple outlet extension leads. If there is hidden damage to the earthing wire of the extension cable, the hazard will increase since in this case the sum of all stray currents from the equipment connected to the same extension cord will be present in all equipment.

Rule 3

Extension leads, even those with only a single socket, should never be used. If you need a longer connecting cable, have your engineering department install one for you.

Rule 4

Damaged connectors, socket outlets and cables must not be used under any circumstances. Do not try to 'repair' them using medical adhesive tape or similar material.

Rule 5

Try to avoid using socket outlets from opposite walls for equipment applied to the same patient. The electrical power distribution network within a hospital will be divided into different sections, each having its own distribution transformer. Depending on the existing load of each of these sections, they may carry slightly different voltages. If such voltage differences are brought to the same patient, a voltage equalization may occur through the patient, who then becomes the 'fuse'. It takes only a small amount of electrical current to produce serious injury.

Rule 6

Pay attention to the cord sheathing and make sure that it is fully anchored by the cord grip inside the plug. Cables as shown in Fig. 2.1 should never be used.

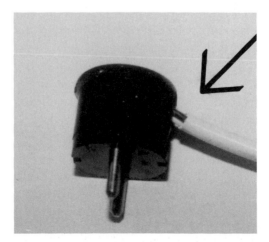

Fig. 2.1   Do not use such cables!

Introduction

Rule 7

Use only those accessories and disposable items that are expressly permitted for the particular equipment in use, for example infusion syringes, tubing and cannulas manufactured by B. Braun Melsungen and by IVAC for infusion pumps manufactured by these companies.

Rule 8

Always make sure that the equipment is correctly reassembled after cleaning, and that accessories are correctly attached or inserted.

Rule 9

Check at least once a day, and certainly before use, whether the equipment is functioning safely and reliably. If you do not, and an accident happens, you may be guilty of negligence if a claim goes to court. Every user manual should describe how to conduct such tests. If not, insist on obtaining this information from the manufacturer before you use the equipment.

Rule 10

Before you connect a patient to the equipment, check when the next safety inspection is due (see the sticker attached to the equipment). Do not use any equipment where this check is overdue. In the event of an accident this could mean serious repercussions.

Rule 11

Assure yourself that the equipment is properly attached to the patient before you switch it on.

Rule 12

Never assume that the equipment is functioning correctly just because it has recently been inspected. Electronic components can fail suddenly and without any warning, and the equipment may consequently not function properly. If the equipment is used over a long period of time on the same patient, perform function tests at least once daily.

Rule 13

After your patient has been connected to the equipment, always check once more that all of the settings are as prescribed by the doctor before switching it on.

Rule 14

Assure yourself periodically that the equipment to which your patient is connected is still functioning correctly. Is there sufficient infusion solution in the bottle? Are the gas bottles still full, and do they have sufficient pressure, etc?

Rule 15

If there is an electrical power failure in the hospital, go to your patient **at once** and check whether the equipment is still functioning properly. It sometimes happens that the emergency generator does not cut in immediately. For patients connected to respirators, external pacemakers, etc., a power failure can be fatal!

Rule 16

Always participate in demonstrations and instruction courses on the correct use of equipment. Make sure that you really did understand all that was said. You must know your equipment if you want to use it safely.

Rule 17

If the equipment is used invasively (for instance for invasive blood pressure measurement, etc.), never touch the patient or invasive metal parts and the equipment simultaneously. You may become a low-current connecting pathway to the patient without realizing it.

Rule 18

Always be aware of the fact that, in the event of an accident, you as the operator of the equipment must take ultimate responsibility. Your superiors may be accused of neglecting their supervisory roles, but the main defendant will be you!

Chapter 3
Examples of Accidents Involving Technical Equipment

Example 1

A child was admitted for treatment to a paediatric ward. One of the treatments involved long-term infusions by means of a mains/battery-powered infusion pump. The child was also connected to an ECG monitor by means of disposable, self-adhesive electrodes to monitor the heart.

When the child had to be moved for examination in another room of the ward, the nurse on duty disconnected the infusion pump from the power supply. This was done by disconnecting the power cord of the pump from the machine but not from the power socket on the wall. The nurse hung the power cord over the housing of the ECG monitor. The infusion pump then operated from the built-in battery. The nurse also disconnected the child from the ECG monitor by disconnecting the electrodes from the electrode cable, leaving them attached to the body of the child.

After the examination had finished, the child was taken back to the room. The nurse attempted to reconnect the ECG electrodes to the monitor but by mistake used the electrical power cord hanging alongside the electrode cable. As a result the child was exposed to the 220 volts power supply voltage and died shortly afterwards.

Applying the basic safety rules to avoid accidents

Rule 1

If equipment is to be disconnected from the power supply, always disconnect the power cord from the wall socket before disconnecting it from the equipment.

If the nurse had applied this rule, the accident would not have happened. This kind of accident is by no means as rare as one might like to believe. Similar accidents have been reported from several countries during the last few years.

References

Bayerisches Staatsministerium für Arbeit und Sozialordnung (1989) Medizingeräteverordnung Informationsdienst 4/89, dated 7 March.

Birkland, D. and Brown, C.E. (1986) Heart monitor mixup kills hospitalized child, *Seattle Times* 4 Dec., p. C1.

Bruner, J.M.R. and Leonhard, P. (1987) Monitors, connectors, and electrocution, *Med. Instrumentation* **21**, 288–289.

DEKRA (1987) Gutachten No. S33/2029/TS 87 43208, dated 24 November.

Katcher, M.L., Shapiro, M.M. and Guist, C. (1986) Severe injury and death associated with home infant cardiorespiratory monitors, *Pediatrics* **78**, 775–779.

Shockloss, W.D. (1989) Better safe than sorry, *Medical Electronics* **119**, 198.

Weiss, T., Böhler, T., Schneider, S. and Linderkamp, O. (1988) Risiken der EKG-Überwachung in der Pädiatrie, *MT Medizintechnik* **5**, 173.

Example 2

In a premature intensive care unit, a premature baby weighing only 1200 g was placed in an incubator. Inside the incubator there was an additional electrical warming blanket which, as was discovered later, was not intact. Furthermore it was not licensed as an accessory to the particular make of incubator. The blanket overheated to a temperature of 40°C, a temperature far too high for the baby, which died after a short while.

Applying the basic safety rules to avoid accidents

Modern incubators are equipped with adjustable interior heating so in this case the additional warming blanket was not necessary. The inbuilt heater of the incubator is set for a certain temperature by the nurse according to the physician's instructions. This temperature is maintained by an integral thermostat, which turns the heating element off as soon as the prescribed temperature is reached. If the interior of the incubator cools off again, the thermostat switches the heating element on again.

Additional warming blankets are not controlled by the incubator's thermostat. In the case under discussion, the blanket had a separate thermostat of its own which did not function correctly and so overheated. The warming blanket had not been inspected and approved by one of the Government testing laboratories, and therefore should never have been used. Here we have a combination of faulty equipment and human failure.

Rule 7

Use only those accessories and disposable items that are expressly permitted for the particular equipment in use.

Rule 14

Assure yourself periodically that the equipment to which your patient is attached is still functioning properly.

If both these basic rules had been applied, the accident would not have happened.

It must be pointed out that this kind of accident is not rare. The international medical press has reported at least 12 such cases during the last 8 years.

References

Brenner, G. and Kindler, M. (1990) Verantwortung im Krankenhaus, *Kranken-haus Technik* **6**.

von der Mosel, H.A. (1969) Fatalities due to overheating of baby incubators, Harlem Hospital Annual Report.

Wolgast, T. (1987) Baby-Wärmematte galt seit langem als gefährlich, *Lübecker Nachrichten* 7 February.

Yamuro, S.K. (1987) Hazards of baby incubators, *Nippon J. Pediatr.* **3**.

Example 3

Two patients died as the result of a mistake made during the maintenance of the central oxygen supply system in the intensive care unit of a university hospital. The engineer responsible for this maintenance had failed to inform the intensive care unit of the impending routine maintenance of the oxygen system. During such maintenance, the oxygen supply is interrupted and the various clinical departments have to switch to bottled oxygen. The sudden pressure reduction within the oxygen supply line was recognized by the staff of the intensive care unit only after the control lights started blinking. Manual respiration was started immediately by the unit's physicians, but two severely ill patients died.

Applying the basic safety rules to avoid accidents

Police investigations revealed that the technical staff were not aware that the intensive care unit was connected to the supply system. All the other clinics had been informed properly ahead of time.

Obviously, the accident happened because of insufficient knowledge on the part of the technical department. However, proper attention to basic rule 14 by the medical staff of the intensive care unit could have saved the lives of both these patients. The rule states clearly 'Assure yourself that the equipment to which your patients are connected is still functioning properly'.

References

Anonymous (1987) Kein Sauerstoff mehr: Tod auf Intensivstation, *Aachener Volkszeitung* 21 March.
Court of Justice Records.

Example 4

A 4-week-old baby was connected to an infusion pump for intravenous feeding prior to gastric surgery. The quantity of solution to be administered was calculated for feeding over a period of 24 hours. However, the infusion pump was defective and the total volume of solution was infused within 19 hours. Although the solution bottle was empty, the pump did not automatically switch off but continued pumping, introducing air into the vein of the patient. When this was discovered by the nursing staff, it was too late: the patient had died from a severe air embolism.

Applying the basic safety rules to avoid accidents

Rule 9

Check at least once a day, and certainly before use, whether the equipment is functioning safely and reliably.

Rule 10

Before you connect a patient to the equipment, check when the next safety inspection of the equipment is due (see the sticker).

Rule 12

Never assume that the equipment is functioning correctly just because it has recently been inspected.

Rule 14

Assure yourself periodically that the equipment to which your patient is attached is still functioning correctly. Is there still sufficient infusion solution in the bottle, etc?

In this example, all these basic rules had been neglected. If they had been applied, the nurse would have realized that the pump did not stop automatically at the end of dispensing the solution and that the warning alarm of the equipment did not work. No safety checks had ever been performed on this equipment. If the nurse had observed the patient at least once every hour, it should have been possible to notice that the infusion bottle was emptying faster than intended. Infusion of air would not have happened.

The accident described happened in Germany. Some years prior to this accident a patient died while being treated with the same type of infusion pump. Expert inspection of the pump revealed 19 safety deficiencies. All hospitals within the former Federal Republic of Germany were informed by letter of the possible risks associated with this equipment, including the hospital where the accident described had happened. Unfortunately, nobody appeared to have taken any notice of this letter and the accident was repeated.

References

Anonymous (1981) Tod aus der Pumpe, *Der Spiegel* No. 18.

Example 5

An accident happened in a hospital where a disposable infusion set was used that was not compatible with the infusion pump. It was pure luck that the patient did not suffer serious injury.

An occlusion occurred within the tubing, and because of the resulting pressure built up within the system the part of the tubing connecting the patient to the pump slipped off. With the type of pump used (peristaltic), the system pressure may get as high as 8 bar before the pump stops automatically and triggers an alarm. In this case no alarm was triggered since the pump did continue to work properly and solution was still being pumped through the system. From the hose, now separated from the pump but still connected to the patient's blood vessel, blood flowed out.

Applying the basic safety rules to avoid accidents

Clearly, the reason for the accident described was the use of the incompatible infusion set.

Rule 7

Use only those accessories and disposable items that are expressly permitted for the particular equipment in use.

Reference

Bayerisches Staatsministerium für Arbeit und Sozialordnung (1990) Medizingeräteverordnung, Informationsdienst No. 4.

Example 6

During the use of a surgical laser in connection with a bronchoscope, first the inner part of the bronchoscope, then the outer shell, and then consequently the bronchotubus, started burning. The patient died from the severe burns suffered.

Applying the basic safety rules to avoid accidents

According to the subsequent investigations, the equipment in use was technically in good condition. The flushing gas used was compressed air.

The accident happened because the surgeon had switched on the laser before the laser-light-carrying glass fibre optic had been fully inserted, so the emitting tip was still inside the bronchoscope. In this case, the surgeon did not follow the instruction manual, which stated: do not switch on the laser before you can see through the observation optic that the laser-emitting tip is in its proper position (i.e. outside the bronchoscope).

Reference

Bayerisches Staatsministerium für Arbeit und Sozialordnung (1989) Medizingeräteverordnung, Informationsdienst No. 8.

Example 7

In a premature intensive care unit, a baby weighing about 900 g was connected to a syringe-type infusion pump. Inserting the syringe into its mounting support, the nurse unintentionally touched the selector switch for selection of the output rate. The set rate of 3.4 cm^3/h was changed to 93.4 cm^3/h and the nurse switched on the pump without realizing this had happened. The entire contents of the syringe (40 cm^3) were injected within 20 minutes into the circulatory system of the premature baby. It is not known whether the baby survived.

Applying the basic safety rules to avoid accidents

Rule 13

After your patient has been connected to the equipment, always check once more that all of the settings are as prescribed by the doctor before switching it on. If the nurse had adhered to this basic rule, the setting of the wrong dose would have been spotted and the accident would not have happened.

Reference

Personal correspondence with the hospital.

Part II
Diagnostic Equipment

Chapter 4
Non-invasive Blood Pressure Measurement

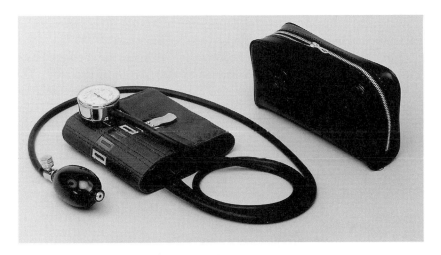

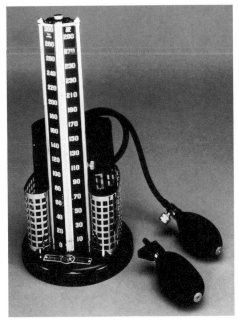

Examples of non-invasive blood pressure measurement equipment

Principle of operation

One of the most commonly applied diagnostic procedures for the measurement of blood pressure uses a pressure cuff. The pressure cuff is applied around the limb where measurement is to be taken, usually the upper arm, and subsequently pumped up with air until the pressure applied is clearly higher than the systolic blood pressure. This causes compression of the artery located beneath the cuff so no more blood can flow through this artery. Thereafter, the pressure from the cuff is gradually discharged. During this period the pulse can be felt distally of the cuff, or, by means of the stethoscope, it can be heard when the blood begins to flow again (when it is known as the Korotkoff murmur). The cuff pressure which is read from the manometer as soon as the blood begins to flow again is regarded as the systolic blood pressure. On further pressure discharge, as the murmur fades away and is finally no longer audible, the pressure now read on the manometer corresponds to the diastolic blood pressure (Fig. 4.1).

It does not appear to be widely known that the width of the cuff should measure approximately 40% of the circumference of the extremity to

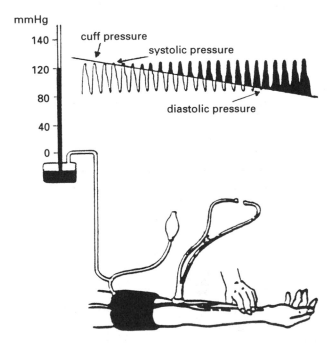

Fig. 4.1   Korotkoff sounds.

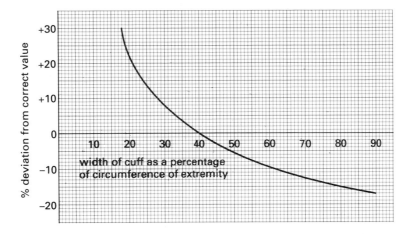

Fig. 4.2

which it is applied. If this is not the case, considerable deviations from the correct measurement value will result (Fig. 4.2).

- If the cuff is too wide, the resulting value of the blood pressure will be too low.
- If the cuff is too narrow, the resulting value of the blood pressure will be too high.

This relation of width of cuff to circumference of extremity applies to all measurement methods in which a cuff is used.

About 20 years ago a new type of equipment was introduced which makes unnecessary the hearing of the Korotkoff murmur by means of a stethoscope, and hence prevents possible measurement faults caused by poor hearing on the part of the examiner). Initially a small microphone was built into the cuff which did hear the Korotkoff murmur. The resultant measurement value was then indicated by the equipment. Such equipment is still occasionally in use.

The more modern equipment uses the oscillometric method. Here, oscillations of the blood vessel wall having different amplitudes are measured directly (Fig. 4.3). These oscillations are then processed by a microprocessor. The conventional cuff is still used; the pressure trans-ducer for measurement of the amplitudes is built into the equipment.

At the beginning of the measurement the cuff is automatically inflated by a compressor contained within the equipment until the artery is closed. On closure of the artery there are still a few oscillation ampli-tudes registered which originate from the proximal part of the artery. However, these are disregarded for the purposes of measurement.

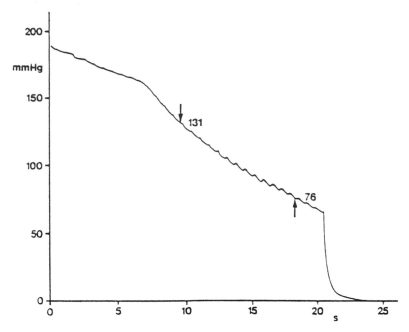

Fig. 4.3   Blood vessel oscillation amplitudes.

After inflation the pressure is automatically slowly released from the cuff. As the cuff pressure goes below the value of the systolic pressure, the artery begins to open up, the oscillations become stronger, and the systolic pressure will be indicated.

As the cuff pressure decreases further, the oscillations become stronger and reach their maximum if the cuff pressure corresponds to the mean arterial pressure value. On further reduction of the cuff pressure beyond the mean arterial pressure value, the amplitudes again become smaller and remain, finally, constant as soon as the cuff pressure is below the diastolic pressure value.

As already mentioned, the use of oscillometry can eliminate subjective influences such as the hearing, vision and sensitivity of the examiner, which may interfere when using auscultatory or palpatory measurements; furthermore the measurement results are more reliable and reproducible.

Also, in contrast to the auscultatory and palpatory measurement methods, the oscillometric measurement method actually permits direct measurement of the mean arterial blood pressure (MABP). During the development of this method, long-term comparative measurements indicated that the MABP values so obtained corresponded quite well to the values obtained mathematically using the invasive method for blood pressure measurement and were reproducible; however, there is not a

100% conformity between the invasive and non-invasive values. However, at only 2–5 mmHg the differences are negligible.

The mean arterial blood pressure is the driving force for a constant capillary blood flow and is hence the most important blood pressure parameter within the arterial system for the judgement of vital functions.

Indications for application of the non-invasive oscillometric blood pressure control are:

- Routine blood pressure measurement in general medical practice.
- Monitoring of critically ill patients if the blood pressure is to be measure within small time intervals (as in surgery, on the introduction of anaesthesia, and in the recovery room and intensive care units, etc.).
- Monitoring of the mean arterial blood pressure if this is an important parameter and the invasive method has to be avoided (as in gynaecology, haemodialysis, etc.).
- In cases in which other, non-invasive measurement methods are unsuccessful or inappropriate (obese patients, premature or newborn babies, etc.)
- Measurement of the mean arterial blood pressure of patients under shock.
- In case measurement cannot be done on the upper arm (as in patients with severe burns, and in surgery in the region of the head, etc.).

Equipment care

Care of the equipment is limited to cleaning and disinfection of the equipment surfaces and the pressure cuff.

Warning: For electrically operated equipment, first disconnect from electrical supply!

To clean the surface of the equipment and the cuff, the low alcohol disinfectants and detergents normally used in hospitals are suitable. Wipe surface with a moist cloth only. **Watch that no liquid flows into the equipment.**

It is important to adhere strictly to the manufacturer's instructions provided for the detergent or disinfectant.

Daily safety check

Most modern non-invasive blood pressure equipment has an inbuilt self-testing function. Where this is not the case and the user's manual does not provide the necessary information, ask the manufacturer for advice on this test.

Application hints

For some of these machines the blood pressure is given in Torr instead of mmHg. (*1 Torr = 1 mmHg.*)

In order to avoid nerve damage and venous congestion (and the possible resultant risk of thrombosis) the following guidelines must be observed:

- If monitoring is necessary over any extended period of time, the measurement interval selected should be as long as possible.
- The extremity on which the measurement is performed should be inspected regularly. This is particularly necessary in the case of automated measurements.
- In order to facilitate the venous backflow, the extremity to which the cuff is fastened should be positioned slightly elevated.
- Do not fasten the cuff too tight. At the non-inflated cuff, it should be possible to put two fingers between the cuff and the skin.
- In the case of extended measurement periods, loosen the cuff regularly for a few minutes.
- The cuff does not have to be placed directly on the skin. For extended monitoring times it is sometimes more comfortable for the patient to place the cuff on top of his or her sleeve.
- If measuring blood pressure at peripheral extremities (lower leg), make sure that these extremities are level with the position of the heart. **Because of the different pressure distribution within the arterial system, these measurement values do not correspond to values obtained by measuring at the upper arm!**
- If the patient is in a sloping position, the hydrostatic pressure has to be taken into account. For each 10 cm above the heart region, about 7–8 mmHg must be added; below the heart region, 7–8 mmHg must be deducted.

Hazards

For the user

- If the equipment is not disconnected from the electrical supply line before cleaning and disinfection, the user may become unintentionally connected to the electricity if any moisture penetrates into the equipment housing.

For the patient

- In the case of electrically operated equipment, there may be a shock hazard if the cuff is not fully dry (the pressure transducer inside the cuff carries electrical current!).
- During the measurement process, the tissues located below the cuff will be compressed. Particularly for cachetic patients, premature newborn babies, and patients with neuromuscular diseases the hazard of nerve pressure lesions exists since the muscular and fatty tissues protecting the nerves are reduced. It is for this reason that in such patients non-invasive blood pressure measurement should be performed at time intervals that are as long as possible. If measurements at short time intervals are absolutely necessary, the risk of pressure lesions should be carefully weighed against the risks of invasive blood pressure measurement.
- Always use extreme care in measuring blood pressure. Faulty measurement results lead to wrong judgement and hence also to wrong therapy including all the possible consequences.

General remarks

Equipment for non-invasive pressure measurement must be recalibrated at least every two years by a licensed agency. Equipment that has been for maintenance or repair must be recalibrated before it is used again.

Further reading

Geddes, L.A. (1970) *The Direct and Indirect Measurement of Blood Pressure*, Year Book Medical Publishers, Chicago.

Geddes, L.A. (1987) The indirect measurement of blood pressure, *Australasian Physical and Engineering Sciences in Medicine* 66– 82.

Hellige GmbH (1989) Zur Blutdruckmessung nach der oscillometrischen Methode, Datenblatt zum Blutdruckmonitor Nl.

Kaspari, W. J. (1990) Blood pressure, *Medical Electronics* **21** (2), 167–170.

Lawin, P. (1971) *Praxis der Intensivbehandlung*, Georg Thieme Verlag, Stuttgart.

Looney, Jr, J. (1978) Blood pressure by oscillometry, *Medical Electronics* **9** (2), 57– 63.

Roloff, D. (1987) Noninvasives Blutdruckmessen, In Freiboth, K., Sonntag, H. and Züchner, K. (eds) *Praktische Gerätetechnik*, pp. 215–219, Verlag MCN, Nürnberg.

Yelderman, M. and Ream, A.K. (1979) Indirect measurement of mean blood pressure in the anesthetized patient, *Anesthesiology* **50**, 253–256.

Chapter 5
Blood Sugar Determination

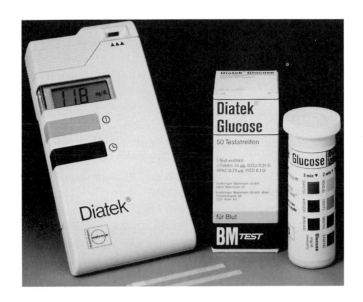

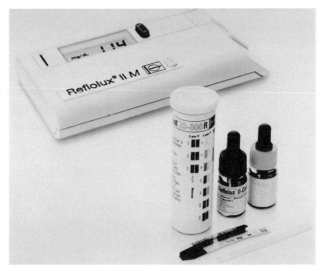

Examples of blood sugar measuring equipment.

Principle of operation

For diabetic patients, regular measurement of the blood sugar values that is as exact as possible is of vital importance. The insulin dosage as well as menu planning for these patients will depend upon these values.

There is a range of simply applied small equipment available for the determination of blood sugar values. All of them work with a so-called test strip. These test strips can also be evaluated without any special apparatus by simple colour comparison with a colour scale printed on the container. However, since very fine colour differences are hard to recognize by the human eye, and since quite a number of people are colour blind to some degree – frequently without knowing it, and particularly since exact measurement is of great importance for the diabetic as a means of enabling the recognition of metabolic aberrations as an early warning, it is recommended that such measurements be done photometrically using the measuring equipment discussed in what follows. An additional comparison of the test strip with the colour scale on the container is nevertheless recommended as a means of checking the proper functioning of the equipment.

The test strips carry on one side a so-called test field, which contains all reagents necessary for the chemical reaction of this test. Among others this test field contains the enzymes glucose oxidase and peroxidase. As the blood is added, the blood sugar is decomposed by these enzymes in the presence of oxygen from the air, which causes a colour reaction. This reaction is measured photometrically by the equipment, and the blood sugar content is indicated digitally in milligrams per decilitre (mg/dl) or millimoles per litre (mmol/litre).

As for all photometric enzyme determinations, exact reaction time, surrounding temperature, and cleanliness of the substrate as well as of the measurement equipment are of vital importance. Measurement equipment and test strips as well as calibration solutions which have been stored in the refrigerator have to be warmed up to room temperature before they can be used. Measurements should always be done at temperatures between 18 and 35°C.

Equipment care

As with all sensitive measuring equipment, blood sugar measuring equipment needs regular care. This includes:

- cleaning the equipment housing using a damp cloth;

- cleaning the test strip receptacle according to the manufacturer's recommendations.

This cleaning procedure must be carried out at least once a week.

Battery condition test

Batteries of such equipment are usually sufficient to carry out about 1000 blood sugar determinations. However, do not rely on the fact that your battery was relatively new. You do not know how long it was stored before you obtained it. Since the batteries of some of this equipment may not be easily obtainable, it is recommended that you purchase a spare battery in good time.

Some of this equipment has an indicator that shows when the battery is getting weak (for instance Diatek of Boehringer/Mannheim: 'Low Batt.', or 'Reflolux II' from the same manufacturer: 'PPP', etc.). If this indication appears, some 20 further tests can still usually be performed before the battery finally becomes dead.

Daily safety check

The function test for blood sugar measuring equipment has to be performed regularly, at least once weekly. Two measurements (low and high value) are made with test solutions (for instance 'Reflolux II-Control') according to the instructions printed on the bottle. If the values obtained during these tests are not within the tolerances given on the test solution bottle, the following should be checked:

- Was the test performed correctly according to the equipment instruction booklet?
- Was the code of the test strip package input correctly?
- Were the room temperature, the temperature of the equipment, the test strips, and the test solutions within the temperature range of 18 to 35°C (temperatures outside this range will cause wrong readings)?
- Was the measuring chamber of the equipment clean?
- Is the battery of the equipment still charged up?

If all these items have been checked and the measurement values are still not within the given tolerances, the user should call the manufacturer for further advice. Eventually the equipment will have to be sent for repair.

Application hints

For blood sugar determination using test strips, use only fresh capillary blood. Venous blood, or blood containing coagulation or glycolysis blocker, is *not* suitable for this test. Also blood samples which have been taken some minutes before the test is performed are not suitable.

Before the blood is taken, wash the hands of the patient using warm water and soap, and rub completely dry in order to ensure thorough cleaning of the skin as well as good circulation within the peripheral capillaries.

In case it should be necessary to use a disinfectant at the point of puncture, **use exclusively colourless disinfectants**. The disinfectant must have completely evaporated before the puncture is performed.

For puncturing, the sides of the finger tip should be used, not the finger tip itself. **Do not squeeze the blood out: it must flow freely!** Discard the first drop of blood (there is the possibility of a wrong measurement value).

If the second drop of blood is large enough, transfer it to the test field of the test strip without touching it with the finger itself. **The test field must be covered completely with the blood**. Transferring the blood to the test field using a capillary is not recommended.

After a reaction time of 60 seconds for the blood on the test field, the blood drop must be wiped off using a cotton swab and only low pressure. For some test strips, the drop of blood is removed using running water. **To remove the blood, use untreated, pure, medical cotton only!** Cosmetic cotton balls or cellulose (paper napkins, etc.) may contain substances that react chemically with the test field and hence should not be used (giving the possibility of wrong results). Remove very carefully any cotton residues left on the test field since they also might influence the measurement result.

The test strip is then inserted into the measuring equipment (test field first), and after another 60 seconds of waiting time (total $2 \times 60 = 120$ seconds) the measured result is indicated by the equipment. It is recommended that the colour of the test field be subsequently compared with the colour scale on the container of the test strips as a counter control. Both values so obtained should not deviate much from each other. The decisive measurement value is the one indicated by the equipment.

Hazards

Wrong measurement results of medical diagnostic equipment which influence the therapeutic measures (in this case insulin dosage) can cause considerable hazards for the patient. It is also the opinion of the author that blood sugar measuring equipment is frequently not regarded as critical equipment, leading to carelessness in its use and maintenance which is quite dangerous.

General remarks

Measurement of blood sugar values should be performed within a temperature range of 18 to 35° and at a humidity not exceeding 85%. Do not expose the equipment to direct sunlight (the author has frequently seen such equipment stored on the window sill!). The equipment should always be stored at least 3 m away from any kind of microwave equipment, diathermy equipment, television sets and radio communication equipment.

The author has observed that the daily safety check as described is rarely performed. However, in the event of an accident, the court will regard this as severe negligence, and will pronounce judgment accordingly!

Further reading

Nöthlichs, M. and Weber, H.P. (1991) Sicherheitsvorschriften für medizinisch-technische Geräte – Kommentar und Text-Sammlung, E. Schmidt Verlag, Berlin.
Stiftung Warentest Eine Hilfe für Diabetiker?, Test 3/86, p. 269.
User's manuals from the manufacturers.

Chapter 6
Electrocardiographs

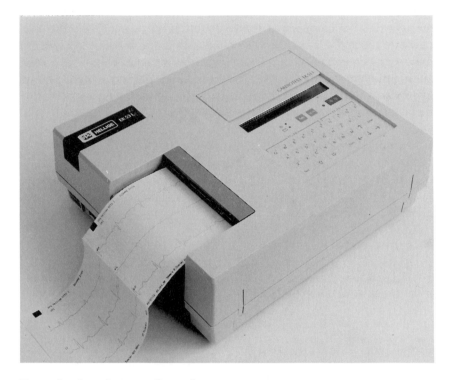

Example of an electrocardiograph.

Principle of operation

In the following the principle of operation of the electrocardiograph will be explained using physiological not pathological electrocardiograms. It is important to realize that the ECG shows only the electrical functions not the muscular reactions of the heart. For better understanding, the different phases of the ECG together with the respective electrical processes are described using a number of drawings in the following.

The cardiac muscle has the properties of (electrical) stimulability, stimulus formation, stimulus conductance, and contractability. From physiology lectures the reader will know that a muscle will react to electrical stimulation by contraction. Normally, the stimulus formation of the heart (pacemaker function) begins within the sino-atrial node and is conducted from there through special pathways, the bundles of His, to all parts of the ventricles.

The stimulus triggered by the sino-atrial node stimulates first the left and then the right atrium and causes their contraction (Fig. 6.1).

Since the electrical stimulus coming from the sino-atrial node flows through the tissue towards the *positive* ECG electrode, it produces an upwards travelling wave, the so-called P-wave, in the cardiogram. Its duration is normally about 0.05 to 0.1 seconds and corresponds to the distribution time of the stimulus wave through the atria. This causes contraction of the atria which now pump the blood to the ventricles.

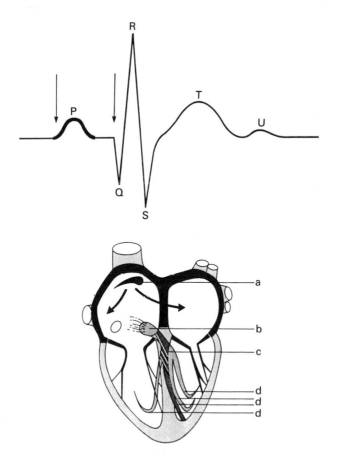

Fig. 6.1 P-wave. (a = sino-atrial node.)

Subsequently, the stimulus reaches the atrio-ventricular node, the only possible location for transmission of the stimulus from the atria to the ventricles since there is an insulating layer of tissue between atria and ventricles which does not conduct any electrical stimuli.

At the atrio-ventricular node, the transmission of the stimulus is delayed for about 0.1 seconds in order to let the blood flow into the ventricles. This delay is seen on the electrocardiogram as a horizontal line, the so-called PQ-interval, also called the atrio-ventricular interval (Fig. 6.2). If the PQ-interval is longer than 0.2 seconds (extended horizontal line), it must be regarded as pathological (atrio-ventricular block).

The stimulus is now transmitted through the bundle of His and then the right and the left bundle branch (Tawara's branch) to the apex. The Purkinje fibres, a fine-meshed network of highly conductive nerve fibres

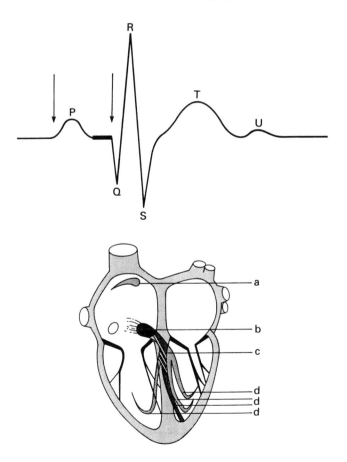

Fig. 6.2   PQ-interval. (b = atrio-ventricular node.)

within the endocardium (the internal wall of the heart), distribute the stimulus through both ventricules. The stimulus is then transmitted from the inside (endocardium) through the myocardium to the outside (epicardium) of the heart muscle which leads to the contraction of both ventricles and hence to pumping of the blood from the heart into the circulatory system.

The depolarization of the myocardium is seen on the electrocardiogram as the QRS complex. First, the stimulus is conducted *away* from the positive ECG electrode by moving from the atrio-ventricular node towards the endocardium, i.e. towards the inside. Hence, we first obtain a *downwards* travelling wave, the Q-wave (Fig. 6.3).

Subsequently, the stimulus penetrates through the myocardium and moves towards the epicardium in the direction of the *positive* ECG

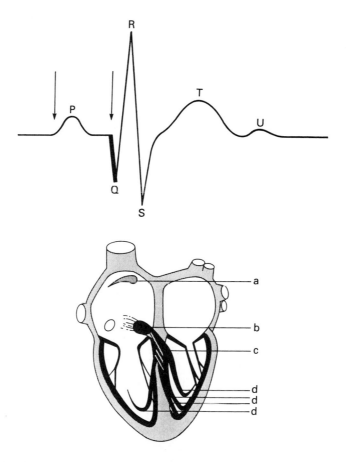

Fig. 6.3 Q-wave. (c = stem of the bundle of His, d = parts of the bundle of His (Tawara's branch) including Purkinje fibres.)

electrode. Hence, we again see an *upwards* wave in the electro-
cardiogram, the R-wave (Fig. 6.4). The subsequent downwards travelling
S-wave indicates that the stimulation has done its job and is fading away.
The myocardium is now fully depolarized.

The ST-interval corresponds to the completed stimulation of the entire
ventricular muscular system. Since all locations within the heart are
stimulated alike, no electrical potential difference can now be recognized: the ST-interval is 'isoelectric' (iso = equal, identical); it is the so-
called refractory phase (refractory = no response).

The T-wave corresponds to the repolarization phase, i.e. the regen-
eration of excitability of the ventricles (the repolarization phase of the
atria coincides with the QRS complex and hence is not visible on the
electrocardiogram). Parts of the ventricles return gradually to the non-
excited condition. There is therefore another electrical potential differ-

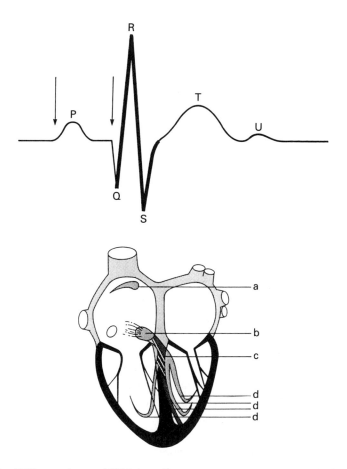

Fig. 6.4   QRS complex and ST-interval.

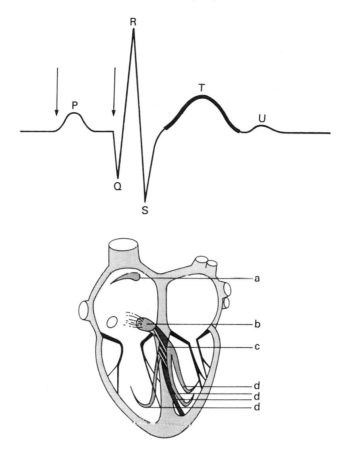

Fig. 6.5 T-wave.

ence the electrical field of which moves towards reformation of excitability, i.e. *towards* the positive ECG electrode. This in turn is indicated
by an *upwards* travelling wave on the electrocardiogram. At the end of
the T-wave, no muscular fibre is in stimulated condition, there is no
longer any electrical potential difference, and so an isoelectric (horizontal) line is seen (Fig. 6.5). Any stimulus in this phase, for instance by
electrical current from outside the body, may cause cardiac fibrillation.
This phase is therefore also called the 'vulnerable phase'.

The TP-interval indicates the relaxation of the ventricles and the filling
of the atria with blood. The U-wave seen occasionally is an electrical
afterflicker (overshoot) without any important diagnostic meaning
(Fig. 6.6).

The electrical signals as described above are received by means of
electrodes attached to the body surface of the patient and are fed into

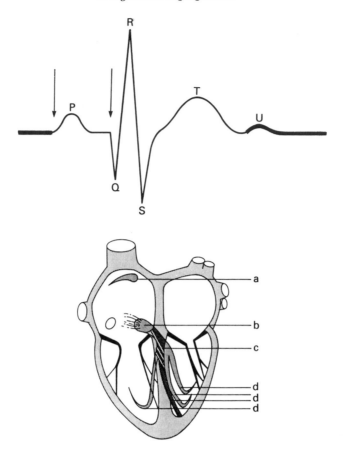

Fig. 6.6 TP-interval.

the electrocardiograph. There, they are electronically amplified and fed to a stripchart reorder which records them on a paper strip (electrocardiogram).

Figure 6.7 shows the different phases of the electrocardiogram.

In addition to the usual resting electrocardiogram as described above, there are a number of additional ECG types of diagnostic importance, as follows.

On the *load electrocardiogram* first the resting ECG is recorded. After this, the patient is exposed to some physical stress (climbing stairs, jogging on a treadmill, ergometer exercises, etc.) and then another ECG is recorded. This permits conclusions to be made about the reaction of the heart to physical stress.

For a *continuous* or *long-time electrocardiogram* the patient is fitted with a portable ECG machine which is carried over a longer period of

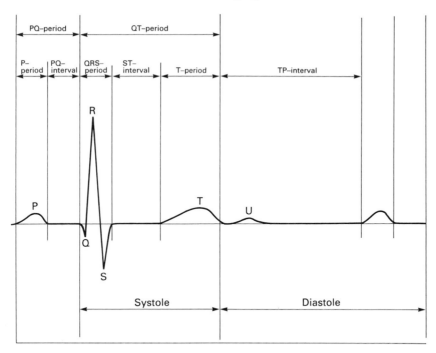

Fig. 6.7 ECG phases.

time in order to record electrical cardiac functions during the patient's normal daily work routine. For this technique refer to the relevant literature.

Occasionally, a *phonocardiogram* is recorded together with the normal ECG. This technique registers the cardiac sound together with the electrical activity of the heart. It serves as an auxiliary aid for the diagnosis of a congenital or acquired cardiac defect (for instance cardiac valve noise in juvenile rheumatic fever, etc.).

In cases where application of ECG electrodes on the skin surface is not possible (severe burns, etc.), as well as for differential diagnosis of transmission defects within the heart, occasionally locations inside the heart (*intracardial ECG*) or within the oesophagus (using a special oesophagus electrode) are used instead.

In intensive care units, constant observation of the electrical activity of the heart is performed using ECG monitoring equipment. These machines are similar to the normal electrocardiographs but they register the ECG tracing not on a paper strip but on a monitor screen. There is provision for the adjustment of certain limits to trigger an alarm in order to alert the nursing staff to the fact that a possibly life-threatening anomalous condition has arisen. Chapter 11 will deal with such monitoring equipment.

Equipment care

Modern electrocardiography machines need little care by the user. Modern technologies, for example thermo writers, make the previously cumbersome exchange of writing pens and refilling of writing ink unnecessary. Some of these old machines are still in use and need such special maintenance, however. In this case, it is important to follow the instruction manual carefully.

If multiple-use electrodes are used instead of the disposable electrodes commonly used today, they have to be cleaned and sterilized very carefully after every use. Also in this case, the instruction manual should be followed strictly.

It is strongly recommended that such equipment be maintained by the manufacturer's service technician at least every 12 months.

Daily safety check

It is particularly important to test the correct functioning of ECG machines daily since only then is a reliable and interpretable recording of the electrical processes of the heart possible.

Most modern electrocardiographs have a built-in self-testing facility which tests the equipment as soon as it is switched on and indicates that the equipment is functioning. In the case of older machines which do not yet have this facility, the use of a 'patient simulator' is recommended. This is connected to the machine instead of a patient in order to do a test run. Such simulators are available on the market, but they are quite costly.

Application hints

The condition and the attachment of the electrodes require special attention since the quality of an electrocardiogram, even with modern equipment, is dependent upon an electrically stable transition between electrodes and skin with a low transition resistance.

To record a normal resting electrocardiogram, the patient should rest relaxed on a patient couch. A relaxed position is particularly important in order to obtain an artefact-free electrocardiogram recording. A suitable arrangement of patient couch and equipment is shown in Fig. 6.8.

The patient couch as well as the electrocardiograph should not be near x-ray, diathermy or ultrasound equipment or near electrical installations with large transformers (for example immediately near lifts, etc.). This is because such equipment may cause interference or indeed eventually harm the patient. The same is true for radio communication equipment, normal television sets, and microwave equipment.

Before the electrodes are applied it is recommended, particularly during the summer months, first to clean the skin of the patient, at least at the points at which the electrodes will be applied, of fat and perspiration secretions using a cotton swab moistened with alcohol. In order to avoid artefacts caused by muscular tension during the ECG recording, the electrodes should if possible be applied at locations having little muscular tissue.

In order to provide as low an electrical transition resistance as possible, even in the case of skin surfaces of different conditions, the preferred materials for electrodes are high grade steel, pure silver, or silver-silver chloride. As a contact medium between the electrode and the surface of the skin, electrode paper, electrode cream or gel are used. Moistened electrode paper is particularly simple to use and provides good results. Also, since it is intended for single use only, it is ideal on grounds of hygiene. It is routinely used in connection with high-grade steel flat electrodes and suction electrodes. Electrode gel and cream are used both routinely and for monitoring, using the electrodes provided for this purpose. For special examinations, for instance in sports medicine or for continuous electrocardiography, disposable stick-on electrodes are used.

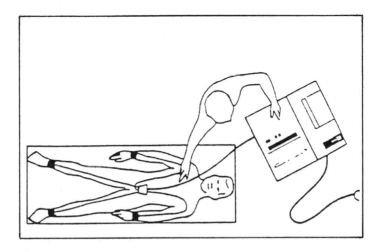

Fig. 6.8 Correct positioning of patient and ECG machine.

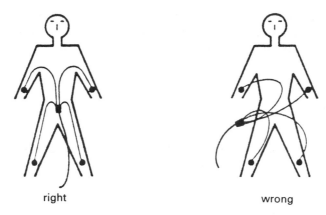

right   wrong

Fig. 6.9 Correct and incorrect ECG–patient cable routing.

After the electrodes have been applied, the connecting cables should be laid out as shown in Fig. 6.9. 'Cable salad' may cause interference and artefacts.

Hazards

There are no hazards for the patient or the user if the equipment is used properly and according to the intended purpose. However, the user is strongly advised to adhere strictly to the instruction manual of the manufacturer.

The issue of electrical safety is certainly important with regard to the electrocardiograph. It is obvious that no electrical current must flow through the connection of the equipment to the patient via the electrodes which could harm the patient in any possible way. For equipment correctly connected exclusively to the body of the patient this is maximally 100 µA during normal use and 500 µA in the event of a fault within the equipment. For intracardial application of the equipment, it is 10 µA during normal use and 50 µA in the event of a fault within the equipment. This requirement is met by all modern equipment. Older equipment should, however, be inspected regularly for safety, at least every 12 months, in order to ensure that it still complies with this requirement.

During practical use of the equipment it must also be borne in mind that the patient may come into contact with external electrical current sources not belonging to the equipment itself. As regards modern equipment, there is no danger since the application side of the equipment (the part to which the patient is electrically conductively connected) is completely separated from all other parts of the equipment.

However, in the case of older equipment (over 15 years old), it is necessary to check carefully that there is no other electrical equipment within reach of the patient which could become an unintentional current source.

General remarks

Only electrocardiographs or monitors that carry the sign ⊣♥⊢ may be used simultaneously with defibrillators or cardioverters.

Further reading

Anonymous (1989) Electrodes – ECG, EEG, EMG, *Medical Electronics* **20** (5), 192–193.

Anonymous (1990) ECG recorders, *Medical Electronics* **21** (2), 122–124.

Conway, N. (1974) *A Pocket Atlas of Arrhythmias for Nurses*, Wolfe Medical Books, London.

Heinecker, R. (1982) *EKG in Praxis und Klinik*, G. Thieme Verlag, Stuttgart.

Hewlett-Packard (1972) *Technician's Guide to Electrocardiography*.

Merz, U. (1989) *Einführung und Interpretation des EKG*, Hellige, Freiburg.

Molz, C. *Einführung in das Langzeit-EKG*, Siemens Publikation No. 117/1800.

Nusser, E. and Donath, H. (1972) *Herzrhythmusstörungen*, F.K. Schattauer Verlag, Stuttgart.

Quiret, J.C., Rey, J.L., Boisellier, P., Lombaert, M, and Bernasconi, P. (1982) L'apport de l'enregistrement lectrographique continu en abulatoire en pathologie coronarienne, *Arch. Med. Coeur* **4**.

Rozanski, J.J., Mortara, D., Myerburg, J., and Castellanos, A. (1981) Body surface detection of delayed depolarizations in patients with recurrent ventricular tachycardia and left ventricular aneurism, *Circulation* **63**, 1172–1178.

Shankara Reddy, B.R., Christenson, D.W., Rowlandson, G.I., and Hammill, S.C. (1992) High resolution ECG, *Medical Electronics* **23** (2), 60–73.

Shockloss, W.D. (1989) Better safe than sorry, *Medical Electronics* **20** (5), 198.

Skordalakis, E. (1986) Recognition of the shape of the ST-segment in the ECG waveforms, *Trans. Biomed. Engng.* **10**.

Vatterott, P.J., Hammill, S.C., Bailey, K.R., Berbari, E.J., and Matheson, S.J. (1988) Signal averaged electrocardiography: a new noninvasive test to identify patients at risk for ventricular arrhythmias, *Mayo Clin. Proc.* **63**, 931–942.

Weiss, T. *et al.* (1988) Risiken der EKG-Überwachung in der Pädiatrie, *Medizintechnik* **108** (5), 173–176.

Chapter 7
Endoscopes

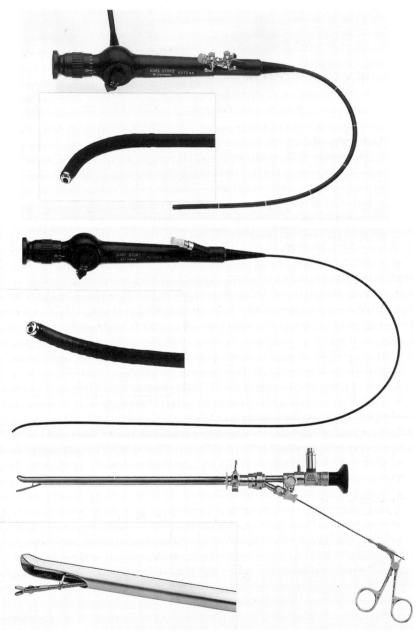

Examples of endoscopes.

The multitude of endoscopes for different applications permits, within the limits of this book, only a general discussion of this type of equipment, i.e. a discussion of its characteristics and handling, which are generally the same for all of these instruments. For specific problems involving endoscopy equipment the reader is referred to the manufacturer's literature.

Principle of operation

Endoscopes are medical instruments that enable the physician to inspect body cavities and to perform surgical procedures in them without first opening them by surgery. Depending upon the location, accessibility and condition of these cavities, rigid endoscopes (for example cystoscopes, Fig. 7.1) or flexible endoscopes (for example gastroscopes, Fig. 7.2) are used.

Basically, an endoscope consists of a rigid or flexible tube in which there is a special optical system for illumination of the cavity and for viewing (with magnification) the interior of the cavity. This tube contains one or more channels for suction, flushing, introduction of instruments, etc.

Endoscopes are very delicate precision instruments which require correspondingly careful and expert handling. Since they are produced from different kinds of materials they require different handling, storage, detergents and disinfectants. The special requirements as given in the instruction manuals must be followed carefully.

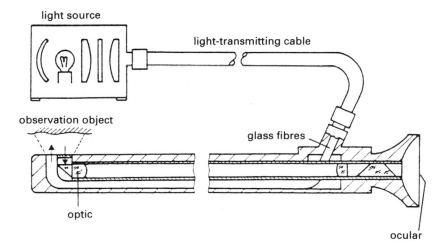

Fig. 7.1 Rigid endoscope (cystoscope).

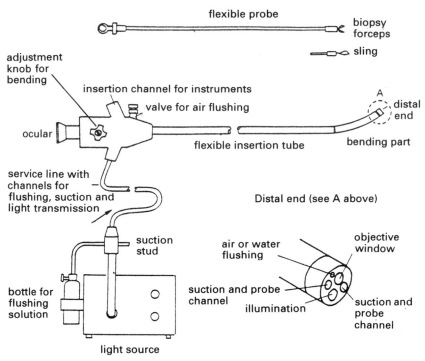

Fig. 7.2 Flexible endoscope (gastroscope).

Equipment care

Endoscopes should be cleaned immediately after each use in order to avoid drying-on of contaminants (and hence difficult removal of them) on objectives and other sensitive components. For cleaning and disinfection the endoscope must be carefully disassembled according to the manufacturer's instructions. It is particularly important that no force be used in cleaning and handling endoscopes (for instance dropping them into the sink, etc.)

The optics are the most valuable and also the most sensitive element of endoscopes and hence require very careful handling. Most damage seen on endoscopes is sustained by the optical system.

Unless expressly mentioned otherwise in the instruction manuals, proceed as follows:

- Disassemble the instrument carefully according to the manufacturer's instructions.
- Carefully remove dirt from glass surfaces using a Q-tip moistened with alcohol. For dirt which cannot be removed in this way, use a

neutral detergent (hand-washing detergent). **Never try to remove such dirt by scratching it off! Optics must never be cleaned using machines or an ultrasound cleaning bath.**

- In order to avoid water spots, use only demineralized or, even better, distilled water for cleaning endoscopes and their accessories.
- When inserting endoscope parts into cleaning and disinfecting solution it is important to ensure that all air bubbles from the cavities of the equipment are removed by agitating the solution or by placing the equipment in a sloping position in order to accomplish complete wetting of all inside and outside surfaces.
- Solutions used for manual cleaning and disinfection must not be warmed above normal room temperature.
- Do not use peracetic acid for cleaning endoscopes since, depending on the material, corrosion may occur.
- After chemical disinfection and cleaning, the equipment must be thoroughly flushed (not leaving any residues) with distilled or, at least, demineralized water.
- After cleaning and disinfection, endoscopes must be carefully dried inside and outside using a cloth and compressed air.
- Incorrect application of lubricants to optics and electrical-current-carrying parts can cause serious faults in the equipment. Adhere strictly to the advice of the manufacturer.
- High frequency surgical electrodes must always be clean and shiny. Obstinate encrustations may be removed using fine emery paper. In doing so avoid damaging or deforming isolation sleeves or handles.
- Most metallic parts of an endoscope (retainer, trocar, trocar sheet, shaft, mandrin, etc.) apart from the optical parts may be steam sterilized separately from each other as with normal surgical instruments. Here again it is important to follow carefully the instructions of the manufacturer.
- So-called fluid-light transmitting cables, i.e. light transmitting cables which contain a specific, optically active liquid instead of glass or glass fibres, must be sterilized neither in an autoclave nor in a gas sterilizer. Here, the use of sterilizing solutions (Alhydex, Gigasept or the like) is recommended.
- Sterilize optical parts according to the instructions of the manufacturer only.
- Special care is necessary in reassembling the endoscope after cleaning. Again, follow strictly the instructions of the manufacturer.
- To clean and sterilize the housing of light sources, high frequency surgical equipment, lithotripsy generators etc. as well as their foot switches, wipe them with a cloth moistened with lacquer-saving cleaning and sterilizing solutions. **Take particular care that no**

solution penetrates into the housing! Before cleaning, disconnect them from the electrical power line.

- Accessible glass surfaces of lamps and condenser systems of light sources may be cleaned with a cotton swab moistened with alcohol.
- Flexible endoscopes should only be stored hanging on the holder provided by the manufacturer.
- To avoid contamination, light sources and the like should always be stored covered with their covering hood.

Daily safety check

In order to ensure that the equipment is in proper condition the following checks should be made before every use.

- Check light transmitter and its cable. Damage (breaks) to the light transmitter can be discovered by holding the proximal end of it towards a light source (a table lamp or the like) and looking into the distal end.

Warning   **Never use the usual cold light source for this test. This light is much too strong and will damage the eye.**

   If black dots are seen within the light beam, this indicates breaks within the glass fibres. Such instruments should be sent to the manufacturer for repair since it is very likely that the light intensity will not be sufficient for endoscopic examinations.
- Check all endoscope parts for external damage and for deformations.
- Check optics for cloudiness. If this cannot be removed by cleaning (see previous section), they must be sent to the manufacturer for repair.
- Check flushing, suction, and instrument channels for obstructions.
- Check all accessories of high frequency surgery equipment for satisfactory insulation. For this purpose there are special testing instruments available on the market (for example from the German company Storz). Acquisition of such test equipment is urgently recommended.
- Check surfaces of high frequency surgery electrodes for cleanliness.
- High frequency surgery generators must be tested according to the instructions given in Chapter 19.
- Check flexible endoscopes (gastroscopes, duodenoscopes, bronchoscopes) for damage due to bites from patients, and open ring folds at the insertion part.

- Check all endoscopes for correct assembly before use.
- Pay attention to special testing instructions as described in the instruction manuals.

Application hints

As mentioned already, endoscopes are very delicate precision instruments. Accordingly they require careful and expert handling. Pay particular attention to the following:

- Because of susceptibility to breaking, the distal end of an endoscope should never be exposed to the effect of any impact or shock.
- Distal movable parts (bending) must be moved only by means of the lever provided for this purpose. Never move them directly by hand at the distal end.
- Never kink insertion parts of the cables of instruments.
- Never over-bend light transmission cables in order to connect an endoscope with the light source. This is particularly important in the case of fluid light transmission cables, which are stiffer than glass fibre cables.
- **Warning: The name 'cold light source' is misleading.** The high concentration of light at the end of the light transmitting cable as well as at the distal end of the endoscope leads to considerable heat development at the focal point of the optic (according to Brubaker (1972), heat up to more than 60°C can develop depending on light intensity). In the event of extended exposure, burns can be caused on biological tissue. Never lay the end of a light transmitting cable on the skin of the patient or on the (plastic) housing of equipment.
- To connect or disconnect light transmitting cables at the light source and the endoscope, grip the cable only at the connector: **never pull at the cable itself!**
- When flexible endoscopes are used orally (gastroscopes, etc.), always insert the mouthpiece in the patient first in order to avoid damage to the endoscope due to biting.
- If high frequency surgery is applied through the endoscope, always use the protective insulation covers for ocular, camera and teacher (second observation ocular) if they are not in plastic housings. All other protective measures as given in Chapter 19 must be applied.
- If laser is used, always wear protective goggles.
- Always apply any additional protective measures as mentioned in the instruction manual.

Hazards

For the user

- Infections because of insufficiently hygienic conditions.
- Burns during use of diathermy and high frequency surgery equipment.
- Burns due to contact with hot parts of the light source and, particularly in the case of high light intensity, the light transmission cable couplings.
- Eye damage when working with laser.
- Explosion hazard when working with high frequency surgical equipment and simultaneous use of inflammable anaesthetic gases. **Observe carefully the 'protective zones' designated by the manufacturer.**

For the patient

- Infection hazard if endoscopes and accessories are not properly sterilized.
- Injury as a result of careless insertion of the endoscope or the accessories or through anatomical anomalies.
- Burn hazard from high light intensity at the distal end of the endoscope (use only for short periods of time, or flush with gas or liquids to cool).
- Burns hazard as a result of damage to the insulation of diathermy or high frequency surgical accessories used in connection with endoscopes.
- Burn hazard during the use of laser.
- Hazard of ignition of inflammable gases in body cavities during use of diathermy, high frequency surgery equipment or laser. Always flush with liquid or inert gases.
- Explosion hazard during work with high frequency surgery and simultaneous application of inflammable anaesthetic gases. **Observe carefully the 'protective zones' designated by the manufacturer.**

General remarks

In this chapter, equipment care has been covered in some detail. Endoscopes are expensive instruments and frequently also have very high follow-up expenses. These are caused usually through repairs as a consequence of wrong or careless handling of the equipment. Better knowledge and, consequently, better care in the use of such equipment can reduce these expenses considerably.

Reference

Brubaker, C.J. (1972) Report of the Working Group on Endoscopy, Committee C-105, American National Standards Institute.

Further reading

Andreas, W.P., Matthies, M., Rodenhagen, P., and Wächter, W. (1993) Gerätekombination in der Endoskopie, *MT Medizin Technik* **113** (1), 18–27.
DIN 58105 Teil 2 (1986) Medizinische Endoskope.
Instruction manuals of the manufacturers.
von der Mosel, H.A. (1987) Hochfrequenz-Chirurgiegeräte, *Die Schwester – Der Pfleger* **5**, 359.

Chapter 8
Monitors – General

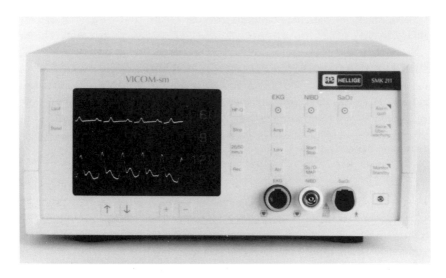

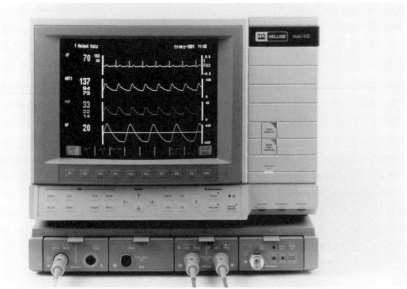

Examples of monitors.

Monitoring of seriousy ill patients in intensive care units by means of electronic equipment is a necessary supplement to first-hand observation of patients by physicians and nursing staff. Without this kind of monitoring equipment, vital data that may change rapidly could not – or at least not with the necessary margin of accuracy – be controlled continuously. Such monitors make possible the timely recognition of life-threatening situations that appear suddenly, and hence enable appropriate therapeutic measures to be taken.

It must, however, be mentioned that 'technical monitoring' of patients can never replace permanent personal contact with them.

Since the technical equipment for patient monitoring is quite costly, it is necessary to consider carefully the parameters that are of life-saving importance for the patient, and only such parameters should be monitored technically. Too much monitoring means unnecessary discomfort for patients because an excessive number of sensors have to be attached to them. It also places an unnecessary burden on the already over-burdened medical staff. On the other hand, too little technical monitoring may be dangerous for patients.

Monitors are diagnostic machines for long-term surveillance of one or several vital functions. Frequently, however, therapeutic devices such as a cardiac pacemaker and/or a defibrillator are also incorporated into the monitoring equipment. A wide range of monitors are available, from simple compact units to complex modular multifunction machines. If they are of modular design, i.e. if they have exchangeable slide-in units for different monitoring functions, they offer high flexibility which permits individual adaptation to existing monitoring requirements. They also provide flexibility so that additional monitoring facilities can be added as required. The different modules can be exchanged from unit to unit without any technical expertise on the part of the medical staff. In the event of service or repair being required (for example for recalibration of a body temperature measuring module), they are just pulled out of the monitor and the rest of it is still usable; only the module is taken out for service, not the entire monitor.

One has to regard the patient and the monitoring system as a technical entity. The measuring chain consists of the measuring object (i.e. the patient), the measuring sensor, the supplying and the receiving cable system, the measuring equipment, and the data indicator. The patient thus becomes part of the measuring equipment, which is also important with regard to the safety measures to be discussed later in this chapter.

The construction of the sensors (patient electrodes) and their optimal application to or inside the body of the patient are of major importance in this measuring chain. The purpose of the sensors is to accept the impulses from the patient and the transformation of these impulses to electrical signals which, subsequently, control the electronic equipment. The function of the measuring equipment consists of acquisition, processing, indication and control of measurement data (Fig. 8.1). **Interference with the reliability of the measurement values indicated is possible at any point in this measurement chain.**

In planning and selecting monitoring equipment for an intensive care unit, the following have to be considered:

- The number of patients to be monitored.
- The space arrangement of the intensive care unit.
- The decision as to whether individual, central or combined monitoring is to be provided.
- The availability of funds.
- Is a local and reliable manufacturer's service available?

For these decisions, the kind of patient is of secondary importance since almost always the same parameters of vital functions are of decisive importance in critical situations. Also for reasons of rationalization, an intensive care unit has to be equipped in such a way that threatening diseases of all kinds can be monitored and treated.

When acquiring monitoring equipment one has to know, too, what is really necessary. Absolutely necessary is the ECG monitor, as a rule including cardiac and pulse frequency. Of only limited importance is monitoring of arterial and venous blood pressure as well as respiratory functions. Monitoring of body temperature is necessary to only a very

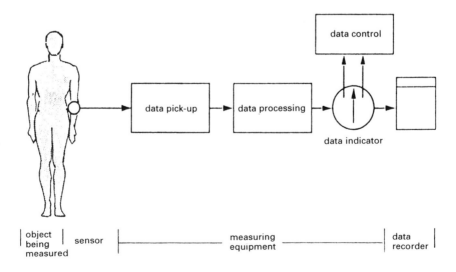

Fig. 8.1 Patient–machine interface.

limited degree. Every one of these monitoring modules has to be equipped with an adjustable threshold alarm which permits individual adjustment of maximally permissible upper and lower threshold values and which sounds an acoustical and/or optical alarm if the set values are exceeded.

However, it is also important to be aware of the fact that not all critical parameters can be controlled by such monitors. Hence, first-hand observation of the patient must never be neglected.

As mentioned previously, the patient becomes part of the measuring chain. For safety reasons it is therefore necessary that the patient always be reliably protected from unwanted electrical currents, including those due to equipment faults. Although modern medical equipment has built-in safety provisions against such currents, special protective measures such as reliable grounding of the equipment and connection of it to a special equalizer ground bus are absolutely necessary. The relevant instructions in the user's manual must be followed strictly. The user should always ensure that the equipment is safe and in reliable working condition before attaching it to the patient. Life-saving and/or life-supporting equipment loses its value if it harms or even kills patients just because of the carelessness of the user.

In the following chapters, the different functional modules of monitors will be discussed.

Further reading

Farah, G. (1989) Patient monitoring trends: from vital-signs measurement to clinical information management, *Medical Electronics* **20** (5), 208.

Moon, J.B. (1992) Patient monitoring outside the ICU, *Medical Electronics* **23** (1), 68–71.

von der Mosel, H.A. (1977) Some common mistakes in planning intensive care units, *Hospital Engineering* **31** (5), 11–16.

Rourke, A.J.J. *et al.* (1966) Details are critical in intensive care unit design, *Hospitals* **40**, 81.

Swan, H.J.C. (1989) Patient monitors, *Medical Electronics* **20** (5), 203–204.

Chapter 9
Monitors for Invasive Blood Pressure Measurement

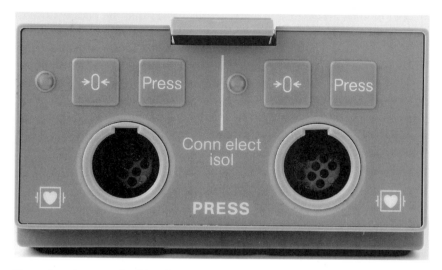

Example of an invasive blood pressure monitor.

Principle of operation

The invasive method of blood pressure measurement is applied if the blood pressure has to be measured at several locations simultaneously (the arterial, central venous, pulmo-arterial blood pressure, etc.) and if such measurements have to be performed continuously over a longer period of time. Particularly in larger hospitals, this kind of observation in patients who have serious circulatory problems is an important routine measure in intensive care units since it provides a basis for suitable and effective therapy. Its objective is early recognition and counteraction in cases of insufficient blood supply to vital organs based on circulatory disturbances.

Since haemodynamic disturbances can appear very suddenly, continuous invasive measurement of the primary circulatory parameters is presently the only method which permits early recognition of dangerous circulatory situations.

The most important circulatory parameters to be measured are:

- *Arterial blood pressure (ABP) including systolic, diastolic and mean pressure values.* Within certain limitations, the arterial mean pressure value is an indication of the blood volume delivered by the heart as well as of the elasticity of the blood vessels.
- *Central venous pressure as a mean value (CVP).* Within certain limitations, here also the CVP can be regarded as a measure of the blood volume existing within the circulatory system.
- *Pulmo-arterial pressure (PAP) including systolic, diastolic and mean pressure values.* The pulmo-arterial pressure is proportional to the amount of blood which passes through the lung circulation.
- *Pulmo-capillary wedge pressure (PCWP).* The pulmo-capillary wedge pressure reflects the final diastolic pressure of the left atrium and is proportional to the blood volume within the left atrium at the end of the diastole. If the cardiac muscle is impaired, it partially loses its elasticity, and the filling pressure or PCWP will increase.
- *Beat volume (BV) of the heart in millilitres and determination of the heart volume in litres/minute.* The beat volume is the blood volume in millilitres pumped out with every heart beat.

The heart time volume is often used as a synonym for heart minute volume or cardiac output (CO). It is the blood volume, in litres, delivered per minute, i.e. BV × cardiac frequency.

Generally, blood pressure measurements are called upon for estimation of the blood volume pumped by the heart. In exceptional cases, however, the relation of blood pressure versus delivered blood volume may deviate considerably. If, for instance, the peripheral resistance is elevated, considerably less blood is delivered by the heart, despite elevated blood pressure, than the blood pressure value measured would allow us to suppose. Information regarding the effective delivered blood quantity can be obtained only by direct measurement of the beat volume and the calculation of the heart minute volume.

It would be beyond the scope of this book to discuss in detail the techniques for placing the catheters. The circulatory parameters mentioned above were described in order to make more understandable what can be measured using invasive blood pressure measurement. The basic measurement principle is the same for all these measurements.

The measurement system consists mainly of a pressure transducer and a catheter, as well as a flushing arrangement in order to prevent any blood clotting at the tip of the catheter, and several stopcocks for zero adjustment of the measuring system (Fig. 9.1).

The essential part of the measuring system is the pressure transducer.

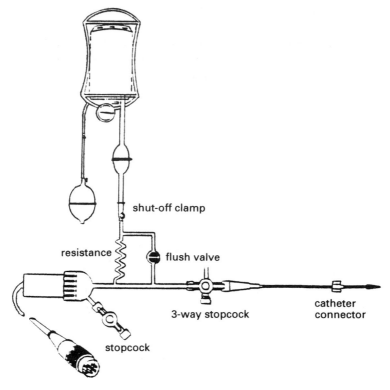

Fig. 9.1 Invasive blood pressure measuring system.

It consists of a chamber partitioned into two parts separated from each other by an elastic membrane. On one side there is the electronic measurement circuit; at the other side, called the dome, is the fluid. To the membrane are attached fine elastic wires which are connected to the electronic measurement circuit. They have an electrical resistance which changes its value if the wires are expanded. If the membrane is vaulted by pressure of the liquid, these measurement wires expand and their resistance becomes larger. Hence, less current passes through the electronic circuit. This change in current passage is proportional to the vaulting of the membrane, i.e. also to the pressure acting on the membrane. The electrical signal so altered is electronically amplified and acts upon a stripchart recorder which produces a pressure curve. By means of an electronic calculator, the pressure values recorded by the stripchart recorder are converted into numbers and appear as a numerical indication on the monitor module.

The complete apparatus is connected to the circulatory system of the patient by means of the catheter inserted into an artery or vein. Hence it becomes part of the circulatory system, i.e. all pressure changes within the circulatory system will cause a pressure change within the measuring system as well.

Since the liquid within the measuring equipment is not flowing but standing, the blood of the patient cannot be used as the head of liquid since it would coagulate within a short period of time and would therefore no longer follow the pressure changes. Instead, physiological (isotonic) saline solution is used to fill the measuring system. It is very important that no air bubbles exist within the system since air is elastic and can be compressed in the event of pressure being applied.

In order to avoid the tip of the catheter which is within the blood vessel being closed by coagulating blood, a slight overpressure is produced within the saline solution. This causes a very small amount of saline to flow into the circulatory system and hence prevents clogging of the catheter tip.

This flushing system consists of an elastic infusion bag filled with physiological saline solution (0.9%) in which by means of a pressure cuff a pressure of 300 mmHg (300 Torr) is produced. It is connected to the actual measurement system by means of an infusion hose having a drop counter bulb and a flow control, and a resistance (as a rule a fine capillary). The resistance (see Fig. 9.1) has two functions:

- Limitation of the flow of the flushing liquid to a few cc/h in order to hold down the measurement error produced by the flushing liquid, as well as to prevent the loading of the circulation of the patient by delivering too much liquid into it.
- Decoupling of the measurement system from the elastic infusion bag which might otherwise act like a large air bubble within the system and might falsify the pressure distribution considerably. By means of an additional flushing valve, a temporary flushing at a higher flow rate is possible.

The entire measurement system consisting of the flushing system, the pressure transducer and the catheter is now filled, free of air bubbles, with the saline solution (Fig. 9.2). Subsequently, the catheter is inserted into the blood vessel.

Invasive blood pressure measurement allows the blood pressure to be measured simultaneously at different points in the circulatory system (arteries, veins, pulmonary artery, etc.) in order to obtain an overall picture of the haemodynamics. Figure 9.3 shows the most commonly used locations for insertion of the catheter for such measurements.

In order to ensure a reliable, faultless measurement it is important to adjust the measurement system to zero before the catheter is inserted. Zero adjustment is the method that takes into consideration the effect of

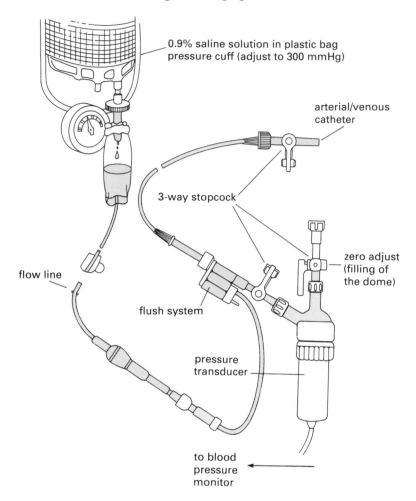

Fig. 9.2   Correct filling of the system.

the atmospheric as well as the hydrostatic pressure on the actual pressure finally indicated.

Atmospheric pressure

The earth is surrounded by a large, gaseous mass, the air. Air consists of different molecules (N_2, O_2, CO_2, etc.), which have a mass and are attracted to the Earth by force of gravity. Air therefore has a weight. Hence, it imposes a pressure on the Earth and on any object on it. The force effected by air per unit area is the atmospheric pressure. It is different at any point on the Earth, and depends upon the altitude and the conditions of the surroundings.

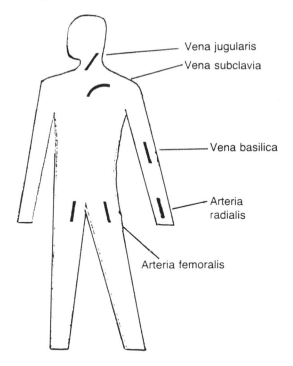

Fig. 9.3 Common locations for catheter insertion.

Physiological pressure is measured relative to the atmospheric pressure, i.e. the pressure values obtained indicate the pressure that exists within the volume or vessel connected to the pressure transducer. After zero adjustment the pressure values obtained do not contain any part of the atmospheric pressure. In order to accomplish this, the pressure indicator is set to zero while the membrane of the pressure transducer is still exposed to the atmosphere, i.e. before the system is filled with physiological saline solution.

Hydrostatic pressure

The liquid contained within the tubing system has a weight too. This weight acts positively on the area of the membrane of the pressure transducer. Hence, a pressure corresponding to the height of the liquid column is added to the physiological pressure. This hydrostatic pressure becomes zero if both ends of the tubing are adjusted to exactly the same level. In this case, the pressure transducer membrane and the catheter tip can be regarded as both ends of the system. Therefore, for all measurements care must be taken that the catheter tip is always level with the transducer membrane at all times. Intrathoracic and intracardial catheters are exactly zeroed if the mean thorax level is used as the anatomical reference point, and the pressure transducer is placed in such a way that its membrane is placed exactly at the same level. In order to determine this reference point sufficiently accurately, a thorax caliper is used. **Zero adjustment of the hydrostatic pressure must be performed before every measurement, and it must be repeated for longer measurement periods.** In addition the measuring system must be switched on for at least 5 to 10 minutes before zero adjustment for the sake of temperature stabilization.

Possible measurement problems during monitoring

Sometimes the blood pressure measurement apparatus of Riva-Rocci (non-invasive measurement) is used to verify the accuracy of the arterial pressure values of the invasive method as indicated on the monitor. This is done particularly if there is reason to question the measured values. Different values obtained by invasive and non-invasive measurement

Table 9.1 Measurement problems that may arise during monitoring, and measures for resolving them.

Measurement problems	Measures to be taken
Thrombus formation, air bubbles, or blood left in the catheter (after collection of blood) will cause excessive impedance	First, remove, by suction and using a syringe, air or particles from the catheter. Thereafter flush the hose using fresh solution
There is a loose tube connection	Seal all tube connections. If necessary replace faulty stopcocks
The catheter tip contacts the wall of the blood vessel, or it forms a node, or an arteriospasm exists	Pull the catheter slightly back or remove it
The wrong system components are used	Shorten the tubing, or replace soft tubing by rigid tubing, or select a larger tube diameter
For the pressure transducer mechanical zero adjustment is necessary	For mechanical zero adjustment always use only the correct technique. An incorrect zero level influences all pressure values but will be more pronounced at lower pressures
The amplifier needs an electronic zero adjustment and calibration	Have zero adjustment and calibration of the amplifier done
Pressure transducer and/or amplifier are defective	Have pressure transducer and/or amplifier replaced

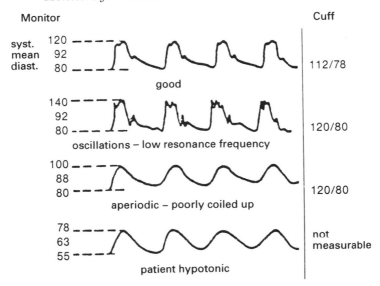

Fig. 9.4 Comparative curves and values of invasive and non-invasive blood pressure measurements.

cause concern particularly if an exact relation of both methods to each other is expected in every situation. For most of the patients monitored one can expect to obtain a value of 10 to 20 mmHg higher if measured with the invasive method than if measured non-invasively. If, however, the values obtained with the invasive method are lower than the ones obtained with the non-invasive method, one must suspect the problems described in Table 9.1.

Figure 9.4 shows comparative curves and measurement values for invasive and non-invasive blood pressure measurement. Typical catheter measurement curves (normal values) for different blood vessels are shown in Fig. 9.5.

Equipment care

The regular equipment care to be done by the user is limited to cleaning and sterilizing the measurement equipment. **Warning: Pressure transducers are highly sensitive devices. They must therefore be handled with care.** Most importantly they must be protected from the effects of shock and from temperatures that are too high. They must never be exposed to temperatures exceeding 45°C. If the pressure dome is removed, the now unprotected membrane is particularly sensitive; careless touching leads to damage to the membrane and hence to the transducer being useless.

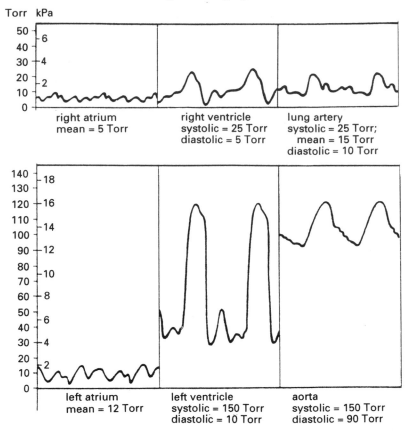

Fig. 9.5 Typical catheter measurement curves (normal values) in different blood vessels.

Careful cleaning and subsequent sterilization of the pressure dome, pressure transducer, and reusable connective tubing is necessary in order to keep them in operational condition and to protect the patients from infections.

Warning: Under no circumstances may detergents containing the following be used:

- perchlorethylene
- trichlorethylene
- acetone
- methylethylketone

as well as other polar-organic solvents such as:

- aromatic hydrocarbons

- chlorinated hydrocarbons
- certain fluorocarbons

Clean the pressure transducer and component parts with a lint-free cloth and 76% alcohol. Use great care when cleaning the membrane of the transducer (without using mechanical pressure) since otherwise the transducer would be damaged beyond repair.

Unscrew (if possible) the connecting cable and fasten the protective cup in place. The cable must be wiped with the usual disinfectant. Here also the substances mentioned above must not be used. Highly concentrated alcohol must also be avoided since it affects the flexibility of the cable.

Protect the transducer during the cleaning process from shock and impact.

All parts of the pressure transducer including the connecting cable may be gas sterilized. First reconnect the connecting cable to the transducer. Before gas sterilization the membrane should be carefully packed into foam material or lint-free compresses. All instructions for gas sterilization must be followed exactly.

All parts belonging to the pressure transducer including the connecting cable can also be sterilized in appropriate solutions. Activated Cidex solution is usually employed. The connecting cable must be screwed firmly to the transducer. **Do not immerse the equipment connector into the Cidex solution. Connecting cables showing signs of damage must not be immersed in the solution. If the equipment connector gets wet, it must not be used again before it has been checked by a service technician.**

Directions for the technician

The resistance between the pressure transducer and the transducer housing must be at least 10 Megohm. Using the transducer at 260 V DC or AC 50/60 Hertz, leakage current must be less than 2 µA.

Under no circumstances must the pressure transducer be sterilized in an autoclave or steam sterilizer since the temperature necessary for sterilization in these machines would destroy the transducer and component parts.

Daily safety check

Most of the new equipment has a built-in self-check. If the equipment does not have this, check the user's manual or ask the manufacturer for the test procedure.

Application hints

When selecting the tubing system for invasive blood pressure measurement the following criteria must be borne in mind:

- The length of catheter and tubing (connecting the pressure transducer) should be not more than 100 cm.
- Use large catheter diameters: not less than 18 gauge/7 French. For children and newborn babies use the largest possible size of catheter in each case.
- Use catheters with a rigid rather than an elastic hose. Materials such as Teflon are frequently too elastic. As an extension tube, do not use the standard, very elastic IV-tube (the usual infusion hose).
- Use tight fitting, not leaking connectors. Stopcocks made of plastic materials are usually more reliable than the reusable stopcocks made of metal. Metal stopcocks develop leaks if they are not regularly cleaned, lubricated and fitted with new gaskets.
- Use the flushing arrangement for continuous flushing in order to avoid clotting in the catheter and the formation of small air bubbles. Even very small blood clots can distort the pressure signal, and small air bubbles can appear in stagnant flushing solution.
- For all pressure lines keep the system as simple as possible. Many additional stopcocks only produce unnecessary confusion and offer good hiding places for air bubbles.

Measurement problems and their handling have been discussed at the end of the previous chapter.

Warning: There is an electrically conductive pathway to the heart through the liquid column and the blood! Blood and all body fluids as well as physiological saline solution are relatively good electrical conductors. Hence, it is important to take care to prevent any electrical currents from entering the body of the patient through the measuring system. Further, the patient should never be earthed in any way (for instance through the metallic housing of the pressure transducer). The pressure transducer must be fastened by means of an insulated (plastic, etc.) holding device. For this reason it is also recommended that plastic and not metallic stopcocks be used.

Fault-free pressure measurement is only possible if the entire transmission system consisting of the pressure transducer, the catheter and the connecting tubing are matched to each other. Diameter, length, durability and elasticity of catheter and connecting hoses influence the pressure transmission behaviour of the system. Once again it must be emphasised: **the entire measurement system including the dome of the pressure transducer must be totally free of air bubbles.**

Hazards

For the patient

- Cardiac fibrillation and other disturbances within the cardiac conduction system caused by electrical current within the measurement system.
- Infections due to insufficient sterilization of the catheter and the measuring system.
- Measurement errors including all diagnostic and therapeutic consequences caused by them.

Further reading

Geddes, L.A. (1970) *The Direct and the Indirect Measurement of Blood Pressure,* Year Book Medical Publishers, Chicago.

Jordan, A. (1986) *Überwachung der Kreislaufparameter, Grundlagen, Schulungsschrift,* Hellige, Freiburg.

Kaspari, W.J. (1990) Blood pressure, *Medical Electronics* **21** (2), 167–170.

Stanley, P. (1967) Monitors that save lives can also kill, *Med. Hosp.* **108**, 53.

Chapter 10
Monitors for Non-Invasive Blood Pressure Measurement

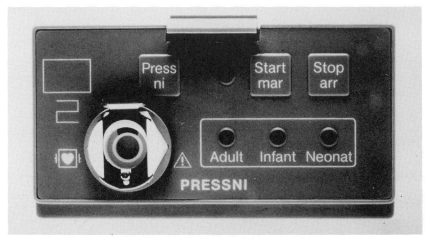

Example of a non-invasive blood pressure measurement monitor.

All details of this module correspond to those of the normal non-invasive blood pressure measurement equipment as described in Chapter 4. The monitor module always uses the oscillometric measurement method. The values obtained are numerically indicated on the monitor.

Chapter 11
Monitors for Electrocardiographic Function and Pulse Frequency Measurement

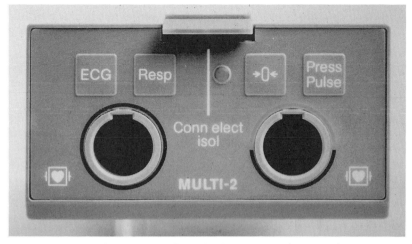

Example of a heart frequency and respiration measurement monitor.

Since the electrocardiogram records by far the most frequently monitored vital function, the electrocardiograph is in most monitors built into the monitor itself. Only occasionally is a special module necessary for this function.

The electrocardiograph has already been described in detail in Chapter 6. We can therefore limit ourselves here to describing the mean differences between a normal ECG machine and the ECG monitor.

Special attention has to be paid to the electrodes which are the first part of the measurement chain. Unsuitable or incorrectly applied electrodes will result in faulty signals which may render questionable the value of even the best monitoring equipment. Therefore, the first issue to be considered is the selection of the most appropriate type of electrode.

With regard to silver–silver chloride stick-on electrodes it is necessary to differentiate between disposable stick-on electrodes and reusable electrodes having a stick-on ring. Silver–silver chloride stick-on electrodes offer a low transit resistance between skin surface and electrode which is reduced still further by the use of contact gel. They also offer the advantage that they are insensitive to electrical voltages from defibrillators since they cannot be 'charged' by external electrical voltages. In normal metallic electrodes the ECG signal will disappear from the monitor screen for several seconds if any DC voltage from a defibrillator were to affect them for even a very short period of time. Hence, monitoring the patient's ECG would be interrupted during this time.

Subcutaneous needle electrodes are pushed under the skin thereby circumventing the high electrical resistance caused by the epithelial layers of the skin surface.

Owing to the very small surïace area of electrodes, electrical burns are possible when there is simultaneous application of high frequency surgery (as in perioperative monitoring) or of defibrillators.

The normal ECG electrodes with stiff connecting cables as are still used occasionally should not be used for ECG monitoring. If the patient moves, they may cause artefacts. The good skin contact which is absolutely essential is only assured for short periods of time with these electrodes, and the relatively long extremity cables render patient care more cumbersome.

Heart frequency is usually monitored simultaneously with ECG monitoring. A special heart frequency module is usually necessary for this.

Principle of operation

The principle of operation of ECG monitors corresponds to that for normal ECG equipment (see Chapter 6). However, here the ECG signal obtained is presented on the monitor screen instead of on a printed paper strip. More complex monitoring equipment offers the additional possibility of paper strip recording. Further, some monitors are equipped with a memory sleeve which stores the signal for the following 60 seconds and stops the signal recording automatically in the event of an arrhythmia alarm. This makes it possible to repeat the signal recording immediately before the alarm was triggered in order to find out what triggered the alarm.

The *heart frequency module* is an electronic integrator which calculates and indicates the mean values of several systoles over a given period of time (usually 5 to 10 seconds). It obtains its signal from the electrocardiograph. An adjustable threshold alarm is built in and triggers an alarm if the set values are exceeded upwards or downwards.

The upper and lower threshold values have to be set for each patient individually according to the physician's prescription.

Equipment care

Except for cleaning the monitor housing occasionally, the equipment does not need any care by the nursing staff. Electrodes and cables for multiple use must be cleaned and disinfected after every use. Residual electrode gel must be removed using warm water and a toothbrush (**never scratch off using a sharp instrument**). Subsequently the electrodes and cables are disinfected in a non-alcoholic solution (for instance Cidex) or in a gas sterilizer. **Under no circumstances use heat sterilization.** The patient cables are cleaned with soapy water first and with a non-alcoholic sterilizing solution using only a moist (not wet) cloth. The cables must be stored hanging, not coiled.

Daily safety check

Since monitors are life-saving equipment, the daily safety check should be performed regularly. Most modern equipment has a built-in self-testing function. If there is none, check the instruction manual or ask the manufacturer how this is done.

Application hints

As already mentioned, the selection of suitable electrodes is of prime importance if a reliable measurement result is expected. No less important is the proper application of these electrodes.

As a rule it will not be necessary to have three channels available simultaneously. For control of frequency and rhythm, one channel will be sufficient. The best recording method presently available is through chest wall electrodes, whereby both neutral electrodes are to be placed at a distance of about 5 to 10 cm and possibly in the direction of the electrical heart axis (Fig. 11.1). However, other means of application are possible. Account must always be taken of the need to ensure that these electrodes are not in the way if resuscitation measures (heart massage, defibrillation, etc.) should become necessary.

If the ECG signal is obtained by chest wall electrodes, the three electrode leads are combined to form one cable. This means that the leads can be short and clearly arranged, so that patient care is not hampered.

For perioperative monitoring the application sites for the electrodes have to be selected as the surgical procedure permits. Particular care in

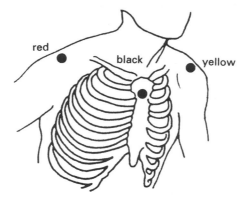

Fig. 11.1   Common placement of ECG electrodes.

the selection of these sites will be necessary if electrosurgery is to be applied. In this case, the following factors must be borne in mind.

- The electrodes must be applied in such a way that the site of surgery (the site of the incision) is not located between two ECG electrodes.
- The ECG electrodes must be applied as far away from the area of surgery as possible.

Figure 11.2 provides examples of the points of application of the ECG electrodes and the neutral electrode of high frequency surgery equipment.

Hazards

Normally, there is no hazard for either user or patient provided the equipment is properly used and the instructions in the user's manual are carefully followed. However, recently there have been reports of accidents, some of them fatal, because ECG electrodes were accidentally connected to the electrical supply line instead of to the ECG monitor. **In accordance with the basic rules given in Chapter 2, if any electrical equipment is removed from the electrical supply line, it must first be disconnected from the electrical wall outlet before the electrical cable is disconnected from the equipment itself.** Reference is also made to Chapter 3, Example 1.

The following possible hazards must also be borne in mind:

- Electrical burns at the electrode site if needle electrodes are used during high frequency surgery.

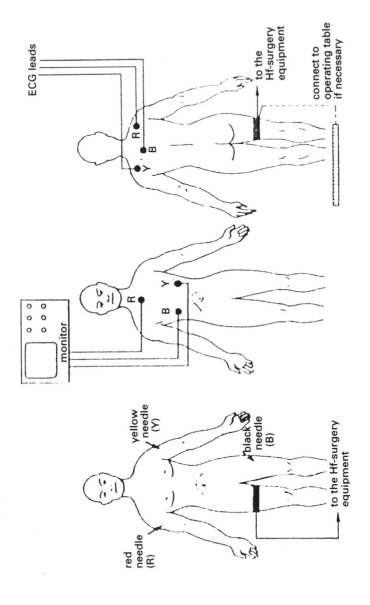

Fig. 11.2 Placement of ECG electrodes during high frequency surgery.

- Electrical burns are also possible at the site of the electrodes if the neutral electrode of the high frequency surgery equipment is wrongly positioned.
- Special care is necessary when applying defibrillation to patients connected to monitors (see Chapter 17).

General remarks

Normally, monitors are used in critical areas of patient care such as intensive care units, operating rooms, etc. Since the life of a patient may depend on them functioning reliably, it is strongly recommended that they be inspection and maintained regularly by competent technical staff.

Further reading

Anonymous (1992) Heart rate meters/pulse meters, *Medical Electronics* **23** (4), 103–104.

Jordan, A. (1986) *Überwachung der Kreislaufparameter, Grundlagen, Schulungsschrift*, Hellige, Freiburg.

Lawin, P. (1971) *Praxis der Intensivbehandlung*, p. 74–77, G. Thieme Verlag, Stuttgart.

von der Mosel, H.A. (1977) Some common mistakes in planning intensive care units, *Hospital Engineering* **31** (5), 11–16.

Nuzzo, P. (1990) Capnography, a standard for the future, *Medical Electronics* **21** (4), 128–129.

Shockloss, W.D. (1989) Better safe than sorry, *Medical Electronics* **20** (5), 198.

Chapter 12
Monitors for Body Temperature Measurement

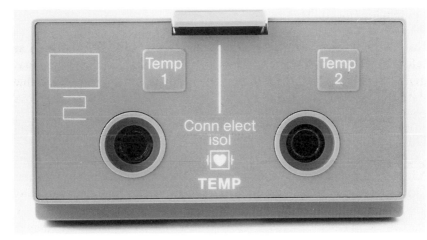

Example of a body temperature measurement monitor.

Principle of operation

The importance of continuous monitoring of body temperature is relatively minor since this measurement parameter usually changes only slowly. Fields of application are therapeutic hypothermia and cardiac surgery involving undercooling and extracorporeal circulation.

The technical principle of operation is quite simple. A thermistor (see also Chapter 14) is attached to a probe and introduced into the rectum or through the nose–throat space into the oesophagus, or it is fastened to the skin surface. Temperature changes of the surroundings cause the thermistor to change its electrical resistance within the electronic measuring circuit. These changes are conducted to the monitor as electrical signals. There, the temperature is indicated numerically in degrees Celsius (°C).

The module is usually equipped with an adjustable threshold alarm which permits individual setting of maximally permissible upper and lower temperature limits. If these limits are exceeded, an acoustic and/or optical alarm will be triggered.

Equipment care

After every use the temperature sensors must be cleaned and sterilized according to the instruction manual and using the detergents and disinfectants recommended by the manufacturer. The connector of the sensor must not be immersed in any of these solutions. Residual adhesive from the tape used to fasten the thermistor to the patient can easily be removed using benzine.

Warning: Thermistors must not be sterilized in autoclaves or steam sterilizers. This would destroy them. However, gas sterilization is permissible.

Daily safety check

Although this test is not so critical for this equipment, it should be performed routinely. Most modern equipment has a built-in self-testing function.

Application hints

For measurement inside the rectum the probe must be inserted via a protective hose. In adults it is inserted about 6–10 cm into the rectum, and in children about 4–6 cm. It is recommended that the connecting cable be fastened to the skin surface by means of adhesive tape.

If the temperature is measured inside the oesophagus, the probe is inserted through nose and throat. In this case it is recommended that the connecting cable be fastened to the skin surface using adhesive tape.

If surface temperature is to be measured, the thermistor should be fastened to the skin (armpit) using adhesive tape. In this case it is recommended that a sleeve be formed with the connecting cable and that this also be fastened with tape to protect it against pulling.

It is not unusual for the body temperature to need to be measured at several different locations simultaneously.

Hazards

No hazards are involved in this kind of measurement.

General remarks

In most countries, temperature measurement devices for medical purposes are required to be regularly calibrated by an authorized government agency.

Further reading

Furler, A.G. (1990) Electronic thermometers, *Medical Electronics* **21** (3), 167–169.

Irmer, W. *et al.* (1967) Therapeutische Hypothermie, in *Dringliche Thoraxchirurgie*, Springer Verlag, Berlin.

Jordan, A. (1986) *Überwachung der Kreislaufparameter, Grundlagen, Schulungsschrift*, Hellige, Freiburg.

Lawin, P. (1971) *Praxis der Intensivbehandlung*, pp. 85–86, G. Thieme Verlag, Stuttgart.

Chapter 13
Monitors for Plethysmographic Peripheral Pulse Monitoring and Pulse Oximetry

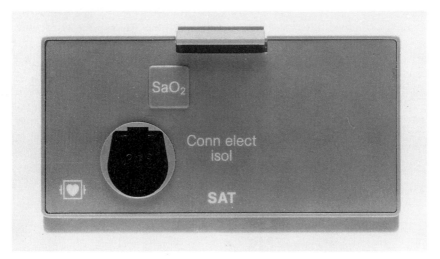

Example of a pulse oximetry module.

Principle of operation

Combining a pulse monitor with a cardiac frequency measurement system and an ECG monitor screen (Fig. 13.1) makes it possible to monitor pacemaker patients properly. If the cardiac frequency of these patients is calculated only by the ECG monitor, the spikes produced by the pacemaker, which will continue to operate, would still show a normal cardiac frequency even in the event of asystoly. In addition, the simultaneous monitoring of ECG and peripheral pulse permits comparison of the electrical heart activity (cardiac frequency) with its mechanical results (pulse frequency). Hence, it enables the early recognition of frustrant stimulation (pulse deficit). In addition haemo-dynamic control is possible with this method.

Photoelectric pulse detectors are used to monitor peripheral circulation by displaying pulse curves. The new infrared light emitting diodes (infrared transmitters) used today instead of incandescent lamps are

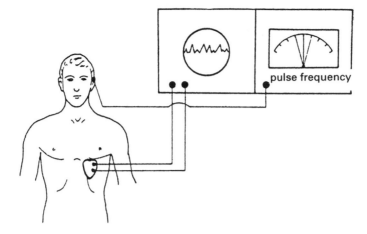

Fig. 13.1   Combination of ECG and pulse monitoring.

highly resistant to interference with the measuring field originating from the surroundings, and they do not cause heat damage to the skin.

The technical measurement principle is based on the increased peripheral circulation during the systole which causes an alteration in the light transmittance of the tissue at the measurement location. The light emitted by the infrared transmitter is reflected by the skin and the blood vessels lying beneath it (Fig. 13.2).

Part of the light entering through the skin surface will be influenced by the continuously changing bloodstream in the peripheral blood vessels. The fluctuations of the reflected light intensity so produced are detected by the infrared receiver (photo cell) as alterations of the electrical resistance, and are conducted as electrical signals to the monitor. There they are indicated numerically as pulse frequency (pulse/minute), or they are displayed as a pulse curve on the monitor screen.

Some pulse detectors use transmitted light (Fig. 13.3) instead of reflected light (Fig. 13.2).

Pulse oximetry serves for the continuous measurement and monitoring of the oxygen saturation (SaO_2) of the arterial blood. It permits

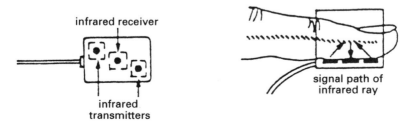

Fig. 13.2   Principle of pulse oximetry.

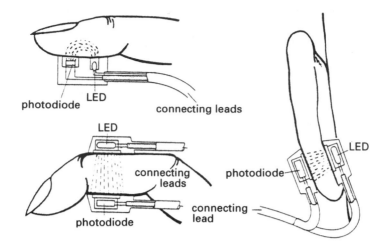

Fig. 13.3 Application of sensor for pulse oximetry.

conclusions to be made regarding the oxygen content of the blood as well as the absorption of oxygen within the lungs, or the internal gas exchange. This enables the early recognition of hypoxia.

Fields of application are child anaesthesia and neonatological intensive care units for recognition of unstable breathing; for neonates for the prevention of sudden child death; for monitoring polytraumatic patients; and in the recovery phase after even short-duration general anaesthesia for early recognition of the disturbances of ventilation and perfusion that are seen frequently. These measurements are also valuable for patients with cardiac insufficiency or cardiac infarction.

The measurement principle is based on the fact that the degree of absorption of the blood at transillumination using selective (filtered) light is a measure of the oxygen saturation of the blood. The measurement is performed using two defined light wavelengths alternating within the red (660 nm) and the infrared (940 nm) range. Within this range, other haemoglobins exhibit the least interference. For differentiation and measurement of concentration of the different types of haemoglobin, their spectral absorption properties are utilized. That is, blue, green, yellow, red and infrared lights are absorbed and reduced differently. One differentiates between pulsating and non-pulsating absorption components. The rhythmically pulsating arterial blood is separated from the constant absorption component and is used for the measurement of the SaO_2. From the quotient of both amplitudes at 660 nm and 940 nm, the SaO_2 is calculated.

In simple terms, the oxygen saturation of the arterial blood is measured using the degree of red and infrared light absorption by the blood.

Measurement errors as well as measurement interferences may be caused by:

- Dyshaemoglobins (methaemoglobin, carboxyhaemoglobin). Particularly in the case of carboxyhaemoglobin (as found in smokers), the SaO_2 value may be elevated by up to 10%. In case of carbon monoxide poisoning, an SaO_2 measurement is no longer possible.
- Movement artefacts by relative movement of the sensor in relation to the tissues.

Empirical calibration of the equipment renders the measurement accuracy of the sensors correct only at their specific measurement site (fingertip, ear, etc.).

Premature babies must always be monitored utilizing the $tcpO_2$ (transcutaneous oxygen partial pressure, threshold 100 mmHg) since a maximal pO_2 (oxygen pressure) alteration results in a minimal SaO_2 alteration (measurement range 90–100% O_2).

Both measurements, i.e. plethysmographic peripheral pulse monitoring and pulse oximetry, are performed using the same sensor. The oxygen saturation of the blood is indicated numerically in percentage on the monitor module.

Equipment care

Photoelectric pulse sensors have to be cleaned **before every application**. Remove connecting cable and connector from the monitor before cleaning. The pulse sensor and connecting cable may be cleaned using a cloth moistened with mild soapy water or an alcohol-moistened cotton ball (70% isopropyl alcohol). Sterilize in ethylene oxide gas at a temperature not exceeding 55°C.

Warning: Under no circumstances must any humidity enter the pulse sensor. To ensure the safety of the patient, never immerse the pulse sensor into any liquids or sterilize it in an autoclave. Before they are reused, pulse sensors must be completely dry.

Always remove the electrical power connector from the receptacle before cleaning and disinfecting the surface of the module. Wipe the equipment with a damp cloth only. No moisture must enter the equipment. All alcohol-containing (up to 70%) detergents and disinfectants as normally used in hospitals are suitable.

Daily safety check

This test should be done before every use. If the patient is to be monitored over a longer period of time, the test should be performed daily. Most modern equipment has such a test function built in. If this is not the case, the manufacturer should be asked for details as to how tests should be performed. For older equipment, the use of one of the so-called 'patient simulators' now commercially available is recommended. The simulator is connected to the module instead of to the patient, and a short test run is made.

Application hints

The pulse sensor is best attached to the index finger or middle finger, the forehead, a toe or an ear (see Fig. 13.3).

Attachment of the ear sensor

- Hyperaemize the ear lobe in order to increase the perfusion. This is done by slightly rubbing the ear lobe, either dry or using 70% isopropyl alcohol. The same effect can be accomplished using a vasodilator cream (e.g. Rubriment).
- Clip the ear sensor to the ear lobe in such a way that the window of the photocell is completely covered in order to avoid weakening the measurement signal by light which does not originate from the infrared transmitter.
- The amplitude of the pulse signal is dependent on, among other factors, the force with which the ear pulse sensor is pressed on to the ear lobe. This force produces a pressure which counteracts the arterial blood pressure. In some of these sensors this pressure force can be adjusted. The sensor should be fastened in such a way that it cannot move but still exerts a pressure as low as possible on the site at which it is attached.
- Do not apply the ear sensor at cartilaginous locations, and always apply it in such a way that it does not press against the head of the patient.
- The use of an ear sensor stabilizer as supplied by some manufacturers is also useful (Fig. 13.4).
- It is vital that the sensor connecting cable is not subjected to any kind of pulling force. A headband as shown in Fig. 13.5 is particularly suitable for this purpose.

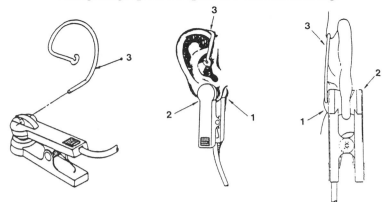

Fig. 13.4   Ear sensor stabilizer. (1 = infrared transmitter, 2 = infrared receiver, 3 = stabilizer.)

Attachment of the finger sensor

- Finger sensors must be cleaned carefully before every use.
- Remove artificial fingernails and nail polish. If this is not possible, the ear sensor should be used instead.
- Hyperaemize the fingertip in order to increase the perfusion. This is done by rubbing the fingertip, either dry or using 70% isopropyl alcohol. The same effect can be accomplished using a vasodilator cream (Rubriment).
- Insert the finger (either the index finger or the middle finger is most suitable) up to the stop in such a way that the fingertip covers the sensor window completely. This prevents light not originating from the infrared transmitter from reaching the photo cell (Fig. 13.6).

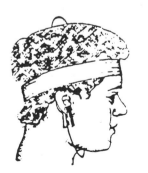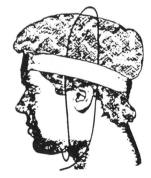

Fig. 13.5   Headband to relieve sensor cable from any pulling force.

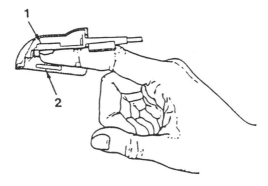

Fig. 13.6   Correct application of the sensor to a finger. (1 = infrared transmitter, 2 = infrared receiver.)

The sensor should be secured at its proximal end using adhesive tape. When doing so be careful not to obstruct the blood circulation. Relieve the sensor connecting cable of any kind of pulling force by forming a loop, and fasten it to the arm using adhesive tape.

During the measurement time, the hand carrying the sensor should rest relaxed on a comfortable support.

For babies and neonates the sensor is best fastened to the feet as long as they are not oedematized. In this case, the hands, the ankles or the calves may be used for fastening the sensor. **It is important to remember that the thicker the tissue is at the location of transillumination, and the less it is supplied with blood, the weaker will be the signal obtained.** Check that the child's circulation is not obstructed after attaching the sensor, particularly on its distal side. Light source and photocell must be placed so that they face each other directly. Ensure that no light from outside can reach the photocell. Always relieve the connecting cable of any pulling force by forming a coil and fastening it with adhesive tape.

Hazards

If the sensors are applied properly, there is no hazard for the patient. **However, make sure that no moisture can penetrate into the sensors!** The sensors carry electrical current which can be conducted to the patient if they become damp or wet, and this can seriously endanger the patient. In the case of patients who are sweating a lot, the sensor should be changed from time to time.

Further reading

Gravenstein, J.S., Paulus, D.A. and Hayes, T.J. (1989) *Capnography in Clinical Practice*, Butterworth, London.

Hänel, J. (1990) Monitoring, *Medizintechnik* **3** (110), 107–114.

Hellige GmbH (1989) *Bedienungsanleitung Servomed, Pulsoxymonitor 236 086 01.*

Jordan, A. (1986) *Überwachung der Kreislaufparameter, Grundlagen, Schulungsschrift*, Hellige, Freiburg.

Lawin, P. (1971) *Praxis der Intensivbehandlung*, pp. 77–79, G. Thieme Verlag, Stuttgart.

Radiometer America, Inc. (1989) Oximetry/bloodgas, *Medical Electronics* **20** (5), 177–179.

Samlhout, B. (1983) *A Quick Guide to Capnography and Its Use in Differential Diagnosis*, Hewlett-Packard, Boeblingen.

Chapter 14
Monitoring of Respiration

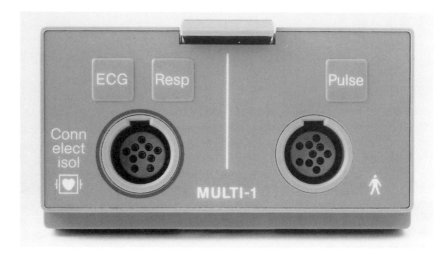

Example of a respiration monitor.

Principle of operation

Monitoring of respiration is of particular importance for patients in whom a sudden respiratory standstill is to be expected (as in severe brain trauma) as well as for patients connected to a respirator. However, in the latter case monitoring is as a rule performed by the respirator.

Usually, two parameters are monitored, respiration frequency and respiration volume.

The monitor functions according to the principle of *impedance pneumography*. According to Ohm's law (see also Chapter 1), the electrical current (in amperes) changes – voltage remaining constant – if the resistance (ohms) through which the current passes is changing. This may sound complicated but it is really quite simple. If two electrodes are applied to an area of the body near the lungs and a weak electrical AC current (10μA, 100 kHz) passed through them, there is an electrical resistance (impedance) between both these locations since skin and tissue do not conduct electricity as well as, for instance, an

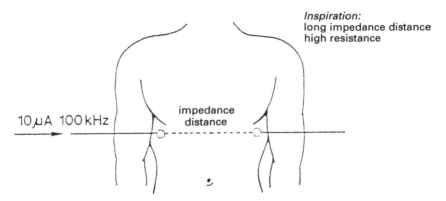

Fig. 14.1 Inhalation – long distance between electrodes.

electrical cable would. During inhalation, both locations of these electrodes move away from each other because of the expansion of the chest, the distance between them becomes larger, and hence the resistance increases and the electrical current passing from one location to the other decreases (Fig. 14.1). Conversely, if both these locations get closer to each other during expiration, the resistance becomes lower and hence more current passes (Fig. 14.2).

This succession of more current–less current is electronically represented in the form of a curve (Fig. 14.3).

After calibration this respiration curve permits measurement of the respiration volume (steeper curve = larger volume, flatter curve = smaller volume) and hence also an adjustment of the setting of a minimal volume which triggers an alarm if this volume is not obtained.

The respiration frequency is calculated, as with the heart frequency, by an electronic integrator from the number of respiration curves per

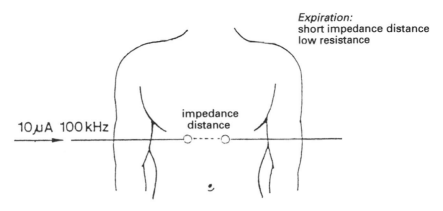

Fig. 14.2 Exhalation – short distance between electrodes.

respiration curve

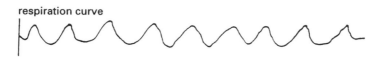

Fig. 14.3   Respiration curve.

minute. It also enables adjustment of the setting of a minimum and a maximum frequency which triggers an alarm if the measured frequency is too low or too high.

At the selected measurement points on the patient's body, electrodes are applied through which the measurement current flows to and from the patient. The most common locations for these electrodes are shown in Fig. 14.4.

For babies, the electrodes should be placed at locations e and f in Fig. 14.4; for adults, placement at locations d and f is preferable. However, observation of the respiration curves enables one to decide which locations will produce the best respiratory signal.

Respiratory signals may also be obtained using ECG electrodes placed on the thorax.

Instead of using *impedance pneumography* as described above, respiratory frequency and volume may also be monitored using a *respiration thermistor*. A thermistor is an electronic resistor that has a temperature-dependent resistance, i.e. resistance becomes lower at higher temperatures and higher at lower temperatures.

The thermistor method is particularly suitable for intubated patients who are not connected to a respirator, as well as for tracheotomized

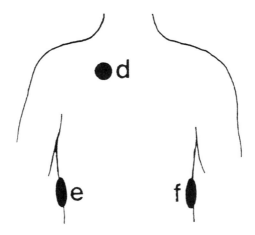

Fig. 14.4   Placement of respiration electrodes.

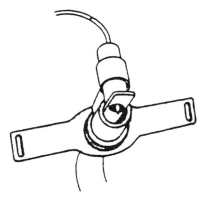

Fig. 14.5   Sensor placement at intubated or tracheotomized patients.

patients (see Figs 14.5 and 14.6). The thermistor is applied within the respiratory air stream. At normal room temperature, the thermistor is cooled during inspiration (room temperature air) and warmed during expiration (body temperature air). The alterations of the resistance so produced by the respiratory rhythm can also be used to produce a respiration curve and for measuring respiration frequency as in impedance pneumography, provided suitable equipment is used.

Equipment care

The module does not need any special care by the nursing staff except occasional cleaning of the housing.

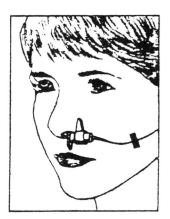

Fig. 14.6   Another way to apply a sensor.

The electrodes for impedance pneumography **must be cleaned after every use immediately after removal from the patient**, as follows.

- Remove the adhesive foil from the electrode and clean the electrode of remaining adhesive by means of benzine.
- Clean electrodes of residual electrode gel using a toothbrush and lukewarm soapy water; **never use any sharp tool to scratch off such residues.**
- Disinfect or sterilize electrodes as described in the user manual. For disinfection use only alcohol-free solutions. **Never sterilize electrodes using steam or water.** Gas sterilization is, however, permissible.

Respiration thermistors are cleaned and sterilized as follows:

- Clean thermistor *after every use* using lukewarm water. It is important to ensure that the connector of the thermistor is not dipped into the cleaning solution. Remaining adhesive tape is removed using benzine.
- For disinfection, any non-alcoholic disinfectant may be used. For cold sterilization the thermistor (**not the connector!**) may be immersed in Cidex solution.
- **Never sterilize the thermistor in the autoclave or in hot air sterilizers; this would destroy the thermistor.**
- Gas sterilization is permissible.

Daily safety check

Since respiratory monitors are life-saving devices, this test should be performed regularly. If the monitor module does not have any inbuilt self-testing arrangement, ask the manufacturer how to perform this test.

Application hints

As with the ECG, the electrode leads for impedance pneumography should be neatly routed. It is important that the electrodes be securely attached and that they will not come off if the patient should move.

In the case of intubated or tracheotomized patients, the thermistor is attached to the tube or to the tracheal cannula (Fig. 14.5).

Another way to attach the thermistor is shown in Fig. 14.6. The thermistor is clipped to the left or right side of the nose in such a way that the protruding tip of the thermistor is within the nasal air stream. The connecting lead is fastened with adhesive tape.

Take care when setting the minimal respiration volume. The smaller the minimum setting the greater the risk of possible artefacts. This may lead to too high a respiratory frequency being indicated, and the apnoea alarm may therefore go off too late.

Minimal respiratory depth must always be newly adjusted after every new application of the electrodes and after alteration of respiratory depth (for instance after remaking the patient's bed).

For patients under assisted respiration the minimum respiratory depth must never be concluded from the respiration curve originating from the respirator since this would not cover spontaneous breaths. Always adjust after observing at least eight breaths of spontaneous respiration.

Check the positioning of the electrodes regularly and watch for artefacts.

Hazards

If average values are correctly adjusted and the alarm threshold is properly selected, and if the electrodes are correctly applied, there is no hazard for either patient or user.

General remarks

Since respiration monitors are life-saving equipment, they should be maintained and recalibrated regularly.

Further reading

Baker, L.E. *et al.* (1966) Physiological factors underlying transthoracic impedance variations in respiration, *J. Appl. Physiol.* **21** (5), 1491–1499.

Bush. L. (1989) Cardio-respiratory monitoring, *Medical Electronics* **20** (6), 83–85.

Geddes, L.A. *et al.* (1962) The impedance pneumography, *Aerospace Medicine* 28–33.

Geddes, L.A. *et al.* (1962) Recording respiration and the electrocardiogram with common electrodes, *Aerospace Medicine* 791–793.

Pacela, A.F. (1966) Impedance pneumography. A survey of instrumentation techniques, *Med. & Biol. Engng*, **4**, 1–15.

Roth, F. (1969) Ein zuverlässiger Respirator-Monitor, *Zschr. prakt. Anästhes. Wiederbel.* **5**, 314.

Valentinuzzi, M.E. *et al.* (1971) The law of impedance pneumography, *Med. & Biol. Engng*, **9**, 157–163.

Part III
Therapeutic Equipment

Chapter 15
Suction Pumps

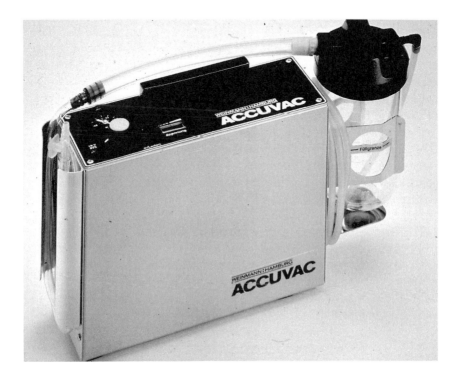

Example of an electrical suction pump.

Principle of operation

Suction pumps are widely used in many hospital departments, emergency and rescue services and others. They are used to suck off blood, secretions, air, mucus, and viscous and solid food particles from body cavities, and they fall under the heading of life-saving equipment.

They generally function by producing a vacuum inside the machine, i.e. a pressure lower than the one at the suction point. This causes air, liquids and other substances to be sucked into the suction hose from whence it is pumped into a connecting vessel.

The vacuum (the under-pressure) is produced either by the gravity of the liquid column contained within the suction hose (syphon drainage according to Bülau); by a vacuum pump; or by vacuum installation in the ward.

Syphon drainage is possible only if the suction hose is always filled with a continuous liquid column, for instance in the case of continuous drainage of the pleura in emphysema or in pneumothorax. In this technique the collecting vessel must always be placed lower than the drainage location, which leads to continuous suction flow caused by the heavier weight of the liquid column in the part of the suction hose that reaches into the collecting vessel (Fig. 15.1). The difference in height between drainage location and collecting vessel determines the degree of vacuum. However, this method is employed only seldom today.

Usually, vacuum pumps are used for suction. Both mechanical and electrical pumps are available. Mechanical pumps are primarily used by emergency ambulances, water rescue stations and the like, i.e. where no electricity is available, whereas electrical pumps are used wherever electricity is at hand. Some of these pumps have built-in batteries and hence can be used everywhere.

The functional principle of mechanical pumps is quite simple (Fig. 15.2). If the bellows are compressed (pump pushed downwards), the air contained inside the bellows is pressed out and escapes through valve 2 while valve 1 (towards the collecting vessel) closes. As the pressure to the bellows is released, a spring pushes the bellows apart, a vacuum is produced inside the bellows which closes valve 2 and opens valve 1.

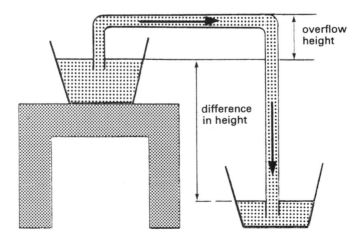

overflow height

difference in height

Fig. 15.1 Syphon drainage.

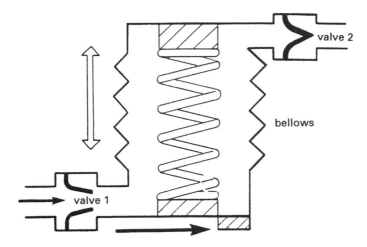

Fig. 15.2 Mechanical suction pump.

Suction is produced within the collection vessel and hence also within the suction hose.

The functional principle of electrical pumps will not be discussed here since there are too many different systems (piston pumps, membrane pumps, vane-type pumps, eccentric pumps, etc.) and their mode of operation is not important to the equipment user. Also these pumps produce a vacuum within the collecting vessel and hence also within the suction hose.

In the case of electrical suction pumps the degree of vacuum can be adjusted by either faster or slower running of the electrical motor or by more or less opening of the suction (aeration) valve on the collecting vessel (Figs. 15.3 and 15.4).

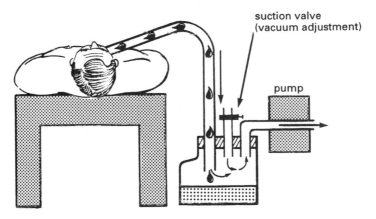

Fig. 15.3 Suction valve of the collecting vessel.

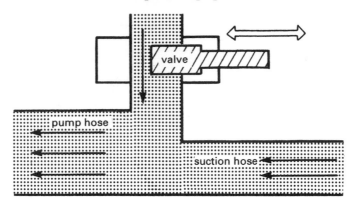

Fig. 15.4 Suction valve.

By opening of the suction valve more or less, the vacuum sucks in a larger or smaller amount of air from the surroundings and hence the vacuum reaching the patient will vary accordingly.

The decisive advantage of suction equipment using a pump is that there is no need for a closed, uninterrupted liquid column within the suction hose as there is for syphon drainage. Even if there are air bubbles, the vacuum is still maintained by the pump. This has the following advantages:

- In addition to liquids, mixtures of liquid secretions and air even up to air alone can also be sucked off.
- Suction is possible from any part of the body where secretions are produced and which can be reached by the suction hose, e.g. body cavities, open wounds, etc.
- Suction equipment can be used immediately and everywhere as long as the necessary source of energy for the type of pump is available.
- A steady and constant flow of suction can be accomplished independently of the position of the patient.
- Suction can be combined with other diagnostic or therapeutic procedures (for example endoscopy) without any problems.
- Hygiene requirements can be maintained by the selection of suitable attachments, for instance bacterial filters, overflow protection devices, etc.

Another method of suction is the use of a vacuum system installed in the hospital ward, or the use of piped air pressure or oxygen.

If a vacuum line is available, the collection vessel is connected to it instead of to an electrical pump. Here also the degree of vacuum is

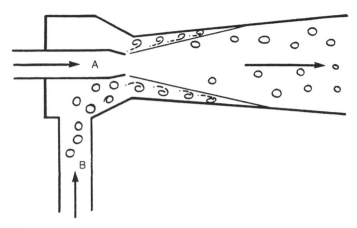

Fig. 15.5 Jet pump.

adjusted using the suction valve of the collecting vessel, or an adjustment valve is installed directly at the vacuum outlet.

If no vacuum line is available, the necessary vacuum may be obtained by means of a compressed air pipe or, if the pressure is high enough, an oxygen line. In this case, a so-called jet pump, also called an ejector, is used (Fig. 15.5).

Air flowing in under high pressure through pipe A expands in the exit pipe (which has a larger diameter) and produces suction in the rear part of the ejector which in turn sucks off air through pipe B. This causes the necessary vacuum in the collecting vessel and hence also in the suction hose. Here again the degree of vacuum is adjusted by means of the suction valve of the collecting vessel.

For long-term suction the use of a collecting vessel with a built-in overflow protector (Fig. 15.6) is recommended. This prevents the

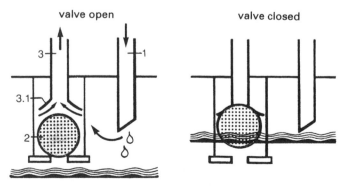

Fig. 15.6 Overflow protector. (1 = connection for suction hose, 2 = float, 3 = connection for vacuum hose, 3.1 = sealing gasket.

sucked-off secretion from entering the vacuum piping and hence contaminating the vacuum system. The overflow protector functions as shown in Fig. 15.6. If the filling of the collecting vessel exceeds a given amount, a float valve closes the vacuum line and stops the suction.

Equipment care

Extreme cleanliness and hygiene are an absolute necessity in order to avoid damaging the health of the patient. All parts of suction equipment which have been in contact with the sucked-off secretion must be carefully cleaned using detergents. Never reuse used disposable items. All reusable parts must be sterilized in the autoclave or gas sterilizer after careful cleaning.

All parts that have not been in contact with secretion should be disinfected with liquid disinfectants or in the aseptor. Electrically operated suction pumps should be cleaned only on the outside with a damp cloth containing disinfectant. Adhere to the instructions given in the user's manual provided by the equipment manufacturer.

If, despite all preventive measures, some secretion has entered the pump, this pump must **under no circumstances** be used again before it has been cleaned and repaired by the technical service.　　.

Where the exhaust air of the ejector passes through one-way filters, these filters must be replaced **after every use**.

After cleaning and disinfection, reassemble the pump following strictly the advice contained in the instruction manual.

Daily safety check

Unless advised otherwise in the instruction manual, check for the following:

- Check visually for external damage. Be particularly careful to check for the completeness of hose connections, and for kinks in hoses or damage to the electrical connecting cable.
- Check that all disposable items used are approved for use with this particular equipment.
- Are all hoses connected correctly, and do they fit the connectors of the particular equipment?
- Are the collecting vessels in good condition? If they have cracks or flaws, the air pressure (vacuum) may cause the glass walls of the vessel to fracture.

- Using installed compressed air, oxygen or vacuum lines, check if pressure or suction is used for the equipment. If pressure is used, an ejector must be used with the equipment.
- Check that the ejector has a new exhaust filter.
- Switch the pump on (or open the valve of the pressure or vacuum line fully), and close the suction valve fully; close the open end of the suction hose with your finger, and using a manometer check that the full vacuum is achieved. After this, adjust the vacuum to the desired degree.
- If a fault is discovered during this test which cannot be corrected by you, do not use the equipment: send it to the technical service.

Application hints

Since suction equipment normally does not have any fault alarms built in, the equipment has to be under constant observation during its application. Pay particular attention that there is always suction, never pressure, within the system. Unwanted pressure may, for instance, occur if the exhaust filter of the ejector becomes clogged.

All hoses must be free of kinks. Check frequently the contents level of the collecting vessel. In the event of overflow, secretion will get into the vacuum line and will cause contamination of the vacuum system.

For long-term use of suction, the collecting vessel and the suction hose must be exchanged at least every 8 hours. The complete suction equipment (including the pump) must be exchanged after at most 24 hours (except in the case of Redo-Drainage using evacuated disposable bottles).

Hazards

The use of suction equipment is not free from hazards. As is usually the case, *lack of attention and carelessness on the part of the user* are the main causes of hazards.

- Use of a suction machine although it has visible damage.
- Failure to perform the daily safety check which would have clearly shown malfunctions of the equipment.
- The required vacuum is not accomplished because one of the hoses does not fit tightly to the connectors, or because one of the hoses is bent.
- The equipment is incorrectly reassembled after cleaning.

- The filter of the ejector is missing. This causes the bacteria contained in the secretion to be evacuated into the room together with the exhausted air. Hence, all patients in this room will be exposed to possible infection.
- If the dirty filter of the ejector is not exchanged at the right time, it may get clogged up. As a result, instead of there being a vacuum, compressed air gets into the suction hose.
- There is an acute explosion hazard if a pump which is not approved for rooms with an explosive atmosphere is used in such an environment.
- Particularly high vacuum may cause severe traumatic damage to mucous membranes or to solid tissues if the suction instrument or the catheter is used incorrectly.
- During suction from the trachea, there is the danger of hypoxia for the patient. Suction should not be performed for more than 15 seconds without interruption. For patients connected to a respirator, special adjustments at the respirator are necessary. Always remember that endotracheal suction is always very painful and unpleasant for the patient.
- During endotracheal suction of an intubated patient, there is always the danger that, in a non-relaxed patient, aspiration of gastric juice into the bronchi triggered by a cough reflex might occur.

General remarks

As with all life-saving equipment, regular preventive maintenance of suction pumps is absolutely necessary.

Further reading

Dick, T. (1985) Suction devices. A guide to emergency field aspirators, *J.E.M.S.* **10**.

Flechsig, R. and Mustermann, R. (1985) Absaugapparate, Schriftenreihe, *Praxis der Medizintechnik*, Verlag TÜV Rheinland, Cologne.

Lawin, P. (1971) *Praxis der Intensivbehandlung*, pp. 222–226, G. Thieme Verlag, Stuttgart.

Otis, O.B. (1954) The work of breathing, *Physiol. Review* **34**, 449.

Chapter 16
Respirators

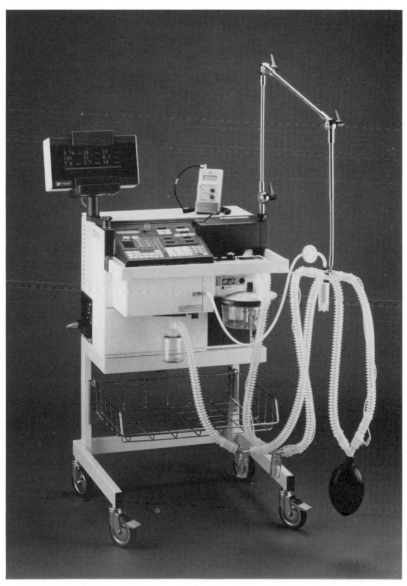

Example of a respirator unit.

Introduction

The subject of respirators is important and difficult. It is important because the application of respirators has caused many accidents worldwide, many of which could have been avoided if the user had had better knowledge of this type of equipment. The difficulties associated with respirators relate to the fact that the information available from the manufacturers is usually insufficient, too technical for nursing staff, and presented unsystematically. The author himself, an experienced bio-medical engineer, has occasionally had considerable difficulty in understanding the user's manuals and principles of operation available to him while writing this chapter, and in selecting the most important and essential information from the material at his disposal. It is hardly surprising that most publications about respirators deal with the physiology of respiration and with respiration patterns, and usually neglect the aspect of equipment function. However, this is the topic of this book.

A multitude of respirators are available on the market. These are produced by numerous manufacturers and the principles of the operation are, unlike those that apply to other technical apparatus, specific to the equipment, i.e. different for each type of machine. It is not therefore possible to use the description of one typical respirator to provide an understanding of all of them as has been done with the equipment described previously. However, it would be beyond the scope of this book to describe in detail all of the respirators available. The author will therefore describe the two most commonly used respirator types in what follows. Cooperation from the manufacturers of other machines may enable the expansion of this chapter in a subsequent edition of this book.

Principle of operation (general)

Artificial respiration means replacing the spontaneous respiration by taking over the work of breathing by means of a respirator. This enables sufficient alveolary ventilation until the cause of the patient's respiratory insufficiency is successfully treated.

We will not discuss here the entire respiratory physiology and biochemistry or the many methods of artificial respiration available; for this, reference must be made to the relevant literature. The subject we have to discuss is medical equipment technology. We therefore have to concentrate on the functions of respiration equipment and its proper application and care. It is safe to assume that such equipment will be applied only by nursing staff who are very familiar with the highly complex field of artificial respiration. This chapter assumes that readers have such knowledge.

Artificial respiration has been known since the introduction of the iron lung by Eisenmenger in Vienna, Austria, in 1929. At that time artificial respiration was applied only in certain acute emergency situations and only in some specialized hospitals. Today it is applied routinely to counteract any respiratory insufficiency, and is used as a supportive measure to maintain life-critical functions in practically all hospitals. For a large number of patients coming from surgical departments to be treated in intensive care units, a respiratory insufficiency exists that requires almost constant artificial respiration by machine.

In artificial respiration we have to differentiate between assisted and controlled respiration.

Assisted respiration is used for patients who still have some respiration activity which is, however, insufficient for the necessary gas exchange. Here, the patient's own existing breathing is used to control the respirator. By application of positive pressure this increases the respiratory volume of the patient. However, assisted respiration is only possible as long as the patient still has sufficient breathing volume to 'trigger' the respirator. At a breathing frequency of 20/min, however, the danger of hypoventilation exists because of the increase of dead-space ventilation. In this case controlled respiration is preferable.

In *controlled respiration* the respirator takes over completely the ventilation of the patient. The machine forces its rhythm upon the patient.

All respirators have one common goal: to provide the necessary amount and composition of respiration gas depending upon the respiration patterns selected at the respirator.

The respiration cycle of a respirator consists of:

- an inspiratory phase
- changeover from inspiration to expiration
- expiratory phase
- changeover from expiration to inspiration.

Inspiratory phase

The kind of inspiratory volume available in regard to pressure and flow volume is partly equipment specific, partly variably adjustable or dependent upon the other adjustments. However, contrary to the normal, physiological conditions of spontaneous respiration, there is always a hyperpressure produced by the respirator inside the lungs during the inspiratory phase.

Changeover from inspiration to expiration

Depending upon the switch-over mechanism from inspiration to expiration selected (called the control), the following basic respirator types can be differentiated:

- Pressure-controlled respirators
- Flow-controlled respirators
- Volume-controlled respirators
- Time-controlled respirators
- Combination-controlled respirators, where several of the above factors control the switch-over.

Pressure control

Switch-over happens after an upper pressure value of the inspiratory phase set at the respirator is reached, independently of the volume delivered or the time passed (Fig. 16.1). Here, it must be borne in mind that the switch-over is not controlled by the alveolar pressure, and that there is the possibility of a considerable pressure difference between mouth pressure and alveolar pressure in the event of high air resistances. Hence, pressure-controlled respirators with constant flow have the disadvantage that, in the event of obstruction of the respiratory pathways, a turbulence with increased pressure head appears ahead of the resistance. This will cause the inspiratory phase to end before a sufficient respiratory volume has reached the lungs.

Pressure-controlled respirators with variable flow can largely compensate for this disadvantage by adapting the flow speed to the air resistance.

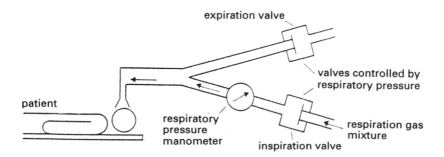

Fig. 16.1   Schematic of a pressure-controlled respirator.

Flow control

The functional principle of flow control is similar to that of pressure control. Switch-over happens after falling short of a preset gas flow towards the end of the inspiratory phase.

Volume control

Volume-controlled respirators switch from inspiration to expiration as soon as a set volume has left the respirator. This volume *must not* be the one effectively applied to the lungs since losses are possible if there are leaks or if there is an increase in volume because of raised elasticity of the hose system.

Pressure-controlled respirators functioning according to the principle of discharge of bellows by pressure built up within a surrounding vessel can be altered to a volume-controlled respirator if the stroke of the bellows is limited mechanically and the reversing pressure is set high. After emptying the bellows and hence also application of the pre-set volume, the pressure will rise quickly to the switch-over point.

Time control

These respirators switch from inspiration to expiration or vice versa after preselected time intervals (by means of an additional pneumatic, electronic or electromechanical timing device), determined by the respiratory frequency (hence also called frequency control) In this case, the condition of the lungs does not have any influence upon the control mechanism; breathing volume, flow and respiration pressure may therefore vary from breath to breath.

Combination control

The different control principles are frequently combined (Figs. 16.2 and

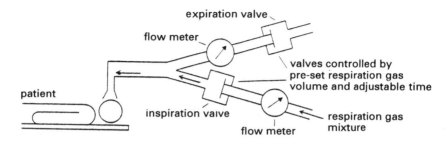

Fig. 16.2 Schematic of a volume/time-controlled respirator.

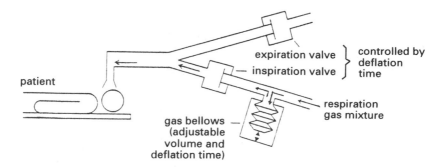

Fig. 16.3   Schematic of a volume/constant time-controlled respirator.

16.3) in order to compensate for the specific disadvantages of each of the different individual systems. In this way, modern respirators offer not only good volume stability but also a multitude of adjustment possibilities for frequency, inspiration and expiration duration, flow pattern, etc.

Expiratory phase

The expiratory phase is, as a rule, passive due to the elastic reactive forces of the lungs and the thorax.

Change-over from expiration to inspiration

Two mechanisms can affect switch-over of the respirator:

● time control: the inspiration starts after the elapse of a preselected time.
● pressure control: the inspiration starts after decrease of the pressure within the respiratory pathways below a preselected value.

Change-over may also be triggered actively by production of a negative pressure (suction) within the respiratory pathways from the patient's breathing. For this type of 'triggering' to occur a sufficiently sensitive inspiration valve is needed on the respirator.

Respirators are driven either *pneumatically* or *electrically*.

Bird respirators of the Mark series (see Fig. 16.4) are pneumatically driven pressure- or time-controlled respirators. Their principle of operation is best explained by means of a respiration gas flow schematic.

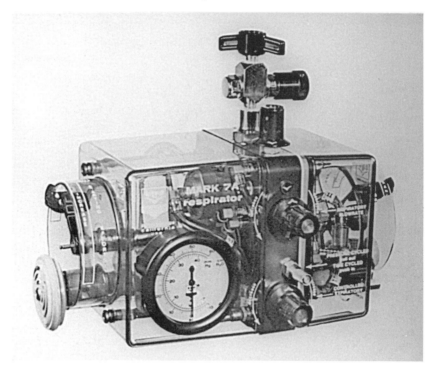

Fig. 16.4 Bird Mark series respirator.

Controlled respiration

During the *inspiratory phase* (Fig. 16.5 (a)–(d)), the ceramic valve (3) is open. This allows the pressure gas (compressed air or oxygen) to flow from the pressure gas inlet (1) via the flow speed adjustment in the following directions.

(In the following, the different gas flow directions are shown separately for simplicity. In real application, however, they happen simultaneously during the entire inspiratory phase.)

(a) The pressure gas flows from the gas inlet (1) via flow speed adjustment (2) and air mixing valve (4) to the venturi tube (5). There the pressure gas is mixed with the normal air of the room which is drawn in through the filter (19). This mixture then passes along the atomizer (main stream) to the patient (Fig. 16.5(a)). Simultaneously, the entire right chamber of the respirator is filled with the compressed air mixture.

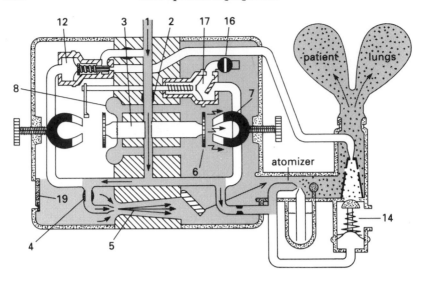

Fig. 16.5(a)

(b)   At the same time the gas flow passes through a stenosis and a
      T-tube to the expiration valve (14) which is held in the closed
      position by the gas pressure (Fig. 16.5(b)).

(c)   Part of the pressure gas passing through a branching-off tube at the
      air mixing valve (4) closes, in the negative pressure chamber (12),
      the valve for the expiratory negative pressure (Fig. 16.5 (c)).

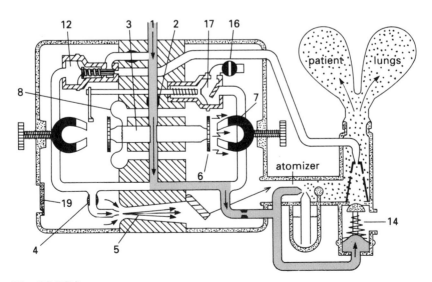

Fig. 16.5(b)

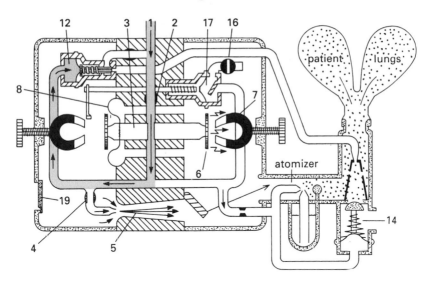

Fig. 16.5(c)

(d) Another pressure gas line 'charges' the automatic cartridge (17) with gas pressure (Fig. 16.5(d)).

As soon as the inspiratory pressure (up to 70 cmHg maximally), which can be adjusted ad libitum, is reached, the pressure to the membrane (8) pushes the ceramic valve (3) to the left side. The right-hand side magnet

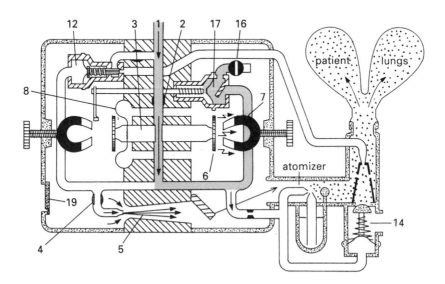

Fig. 16.5(d)

Therapeutic Equipment

(7) holds the right-hand side metal plate (6) until the selected pressure is reached. The desired inspiratory end-pressure is set by adjusting the distance of the right-hand side magnet from the metal plate by means of the inspiratory end-pressure adjustment. The adjusted pressure is indicated by the pressure manometer on the front side of the respirator. This also makes it possible to recognize any resistances that may exist within the respiratory pathways.

Adjustment of the inspiratory end pressure does not set the volume as well. This happens in combination with the flow inspired.

As soon as the preselected end pressure is reached, the respirator switches automatically to expiration (Fig. 16.6).

During the expiratory phase (Fig. 16.6), the pressure gas inlet (1) is closed by the ceramic valve the metal plate of which has been pulled by the magnet to the left-hand side (3). The pressure within the system (right half of the chamber) is exhausted via the atomizer. The left-hand metal plate of the ceramic valve (9) is held in this expiratory position by means of the left-hand magnet (10).

Through the negative generator (11), compressed air now streams through the value in the negative pressure chamber (12) to the negative venturi tube (13). This causes an under-pressure within the expiratory circulation. The expiration valve (14) opens. A relief valve (15) closes the inspiration venturi tube (5) and thereby prevents re-breathing into the system. This pneumatically operated valve also brings about absorption of pressure waves caused by obstructions and slows down

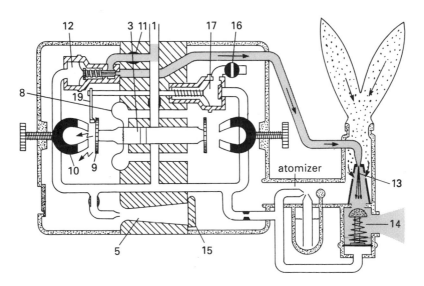

Fig. 16.6

the flow speed hence preventing premature switch-over of the respirator in the event of turbulence.

The needle valve (described as 'automatic' in the user's manual; here labelled (16)) discharges the pressure stored during inspiration within the cartridge (17) which causes the driving rod (18), driven now by the force of a spring, to move towards the right-hand side, touching the left-hand metal plate (9) with a bracket and pushing it, together with the ceramic valve (3) towards the right-hand side (inspiration position).

Assisted respiration

If the needle valve (16) is closed (as shown in Fig. 16.6), the respirator works as an *assistor*. Inspiration by the patient causes the production of an under-pressure within the right-hand side of the chamber of the respirator which will affect the membrane (8) and pull the left hand metal plate (9) of the ceramic valve (3) out of the field of force of the left magnet (10). The ceramic valve, together with the membrane and both metal plates, is pushed to the right into the position of the inspiratory phase. The inspiratory phase functions in the same way as in controlled respiration.

The distance of the magnet (7) to the metal plate (6) adjusts the *end-inspiratory pressure*, and the distance of the magnet (10) to the metal plate (9) adjusts the *sensitivity* of the respirator.

The shorter the distances of the metal plates (6 and 9) to their respective magnets (7 and 10), the stronger is the magnetic force acting on the plates, and the higher will be the end-inspiratory pressure.

Draeger Evita intensive care ventilator: operating principles

The Draeger intensive care ventilator (Fig. 16.7) is an electrically driven time-controlled constant volume respirator for adults and children with a respiratory volume of 50 cc and up. It is designed for:

- controlled, assisted, artificial respiration (IPPV and IPPV/Assist),
- synchronized, intermittent, mandatory assisted respiration (SIMV), and
- mandatory minute volume ventilation (MMV),

and for:

- spontaneous breathing with positive respiratory pathway pressure (CPAP), and
- assistance of spontaneous breathing (ASB).

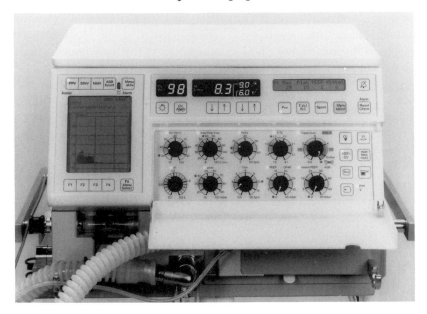

Fig. 16.7   Draeger Evita intensive care ventilator.

The principle of operation is best explained using a respiratory gas flow schematic diagram (Fig. 16.8) together with a photograph of the operational controls (Fig. 16.9).

The basic electro-pneumatic element of the Evita ventilator is the pair of servo valves 7 and 8 (see Fig. 16.8) which are controlled by several adjustment knobs (see Fig. 16.9):

- By opening one of the two valves more or less, the O_2 concentration of the respiratory gas mixture is adjusted according to the setting of knob 1.7.
- By opening both valves more or less, the tidal volume V_T in mandatory respiration is adjusted according to the setting of knob 1.8.
- By opening of both valves more or less, the maximal inspiratory flow V_{max} is limited according to the adjustment of knob 1.9.
- By closing both valves, the inspiratory pressure, as soon as this is obtained, is limited according to the setting of knob 1.10.
- According to the setting of knob 1.11, the opening and closing of both valves determines the time intervals and hence the respiratory frequency.
- At respiration pattern SIMV the valve pair determines for the IFM respiration frequency how often per minute it will open according to the setting of knob 1.12.

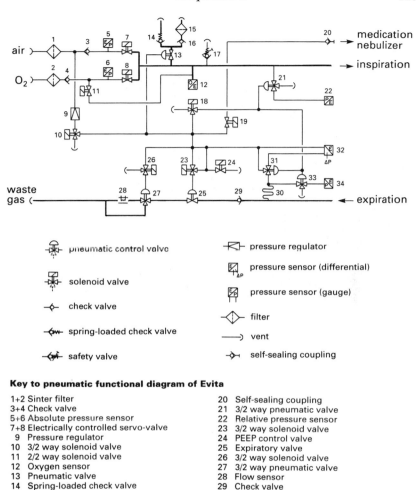

air)

O₂)

medication nebulizer

inspiration

waste gas (

expiration

pneumatic control valve

solenoid valve

check valve

spring-loaded check valve

safety valve

pressure regulator

pressure sensor (differential)

pressure sensor (gauge)

filter

vent

self-sealing coupling

Key to pneumatic functional diagram of Evita

1+2 Sinter filter
3+4 Check valve
5+6 Absolute pressure sensor
7+8 Electrically controlled servo-valve
 9 Pressure regulator
10 3/2 way solenoid valve
11 2/2 way solenoid valve
12 Oxygen sensor
13 Pneumatic valve
14 Spring-loaded check valve
15 Ambient-air filter
16 Check valve
17 Safety valve
18 3/2 way solenoid valve
19 2/2 way solenoid valve

20 Self-sealing coupling
21 3/2 way pneumatic valve
22 Relative pressure sensor
23 3/2 way solenoid valve
24 PEEP control valve
25 Expiratory valve
26 3/2 way solenoid valve
27 3/2 way pneumatic valve
28 Flow sensor
29 Check valve
30 Bacterial trap
31 3/2 way pneumatic valve
32 Differential pressure sensor
33 3/2 way pneumatic valve
34 Relative pressure sensor (guage)

Fig. 16.8 Air flow scheme of the Evita ventilator and explanation of symbols.

Gas flow (general)

Figure 16.10 represents gas flow in diagrammatic form. The pressure gases O₂ (– – – –) and air (- - - - -) from the central gas supply line or from gas bottles are cleaned in filters 1 and 2 and flow through the check valves 3 and 4 to the mixing system. This consists of the absolute pressure sensors 5 and 6 and the electrically controlled servo valves 7 and 8 which adjust gas concentration and flow dosage.

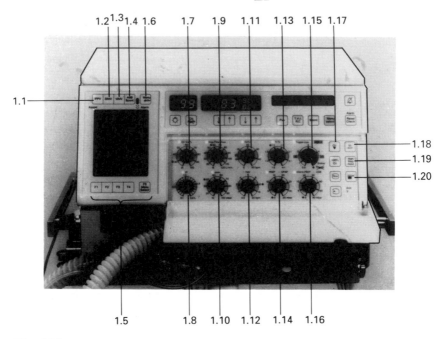

Fig. 16.9

Check valves 3 and 4 prevent a reflux of gas back to the central gas supply line, and hence possible spreading of infection.

Between filter 1 and check valve 3, compressed air is diverted and is adjusted to a given pressure by the pressure regulator 9 and thereafter delivered through the magnet valve 10 to the servo system. Part of the compressed oxygen is diverted between check valve 4 and the absolute

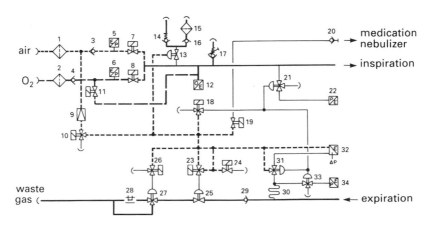

Fig. 16.10

pressure sensor 6, and is delivered through the magnet valve 11 to the O_2 measurement device of oxygen sensor 12.

Safety devices

In the event of failure of the compressed air supply, pneumatic valve 13 is vented through magnet valve 10 which opens, enabling room air to be drawn in. Room air is cleaned by filter 15; the spring-loaded check valve 14 prevents back-breathing.

Over-pressure is reduced through pneumatic valve 13 and check valve 14.

Controlled breathing

Inspiration (Fig. 16.11)

During active inspiration electrically controlled servo valves 7 and 8 deliver a gas flow of defined magnitude and defined O_2 concentration to the patient. The O_2 concentration is constantly monitored by the O_2 measuring device (12).

Safety valve 17 limits the respiratory pressure; if it becomes too high, this valve opens and discharges the over-pressure.

During the inspiratory phase, the expiration valve 25 keeps the expiration line closed. After completion of active inspiration, both servo valves 7 and 8 close.

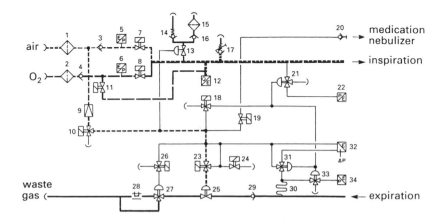

Fig. 16.11

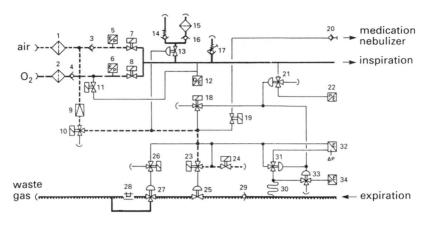

Fig. 16.12

Expiration (Fig. 16.12)

Selenoid valve 23 and positive end expiratory pressure (PEEP) valve 24 open, the control pressure at the expiration valve 25 is discharged, and the valve opens. The expiration gas (▬▬▬) goes through check valve 29, expiration valve 25, pneumatic valve 27, and flow sensor 28 to the waste gas nozzle. Check valve 29 prevents re-inspiration of the waste gas. PEEP valve 24 produces a pressure which acts on the control side of the expiration valve 25 and builds up a PEEP or intermittent PEEP within the respiratory system.

Spontaneous breathing

Inspiration (Fig. 16.13)

The control pressure produced at the PEEP control valve 24 acts through the magnet valve 23 on the control side of expiration valve 25, closes it and builds up a continuous positive respiratory pressure. The inspiration efforts of the patient produce an under-pressure which is measured through the bacterial trap 30 and the pneumatic valve 31 on the differential pressure sensor.

The servo valve pair 7 and 8 now deliver a flow which is proportional to the pressure difference and corresponds to the momentary volume requirement of the patient. As soon as this volume requirement is met and the pressure difference goes towards zero, both servo valves 7 and 8 reduce their gas delivery automatically.

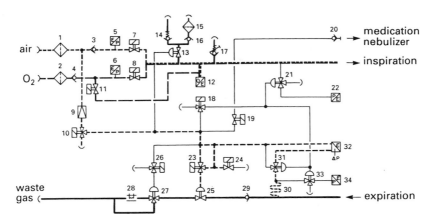

Fig. 16.13

Expiration (Fig. 16.14)

Expiration takes place through expiration valve 25.

Measurement of artificial respiration parameters (Fig. 16.15)

Oxygen concentration

The oxygen concentration of the respiration gas is measured by oxygen sensor 12.

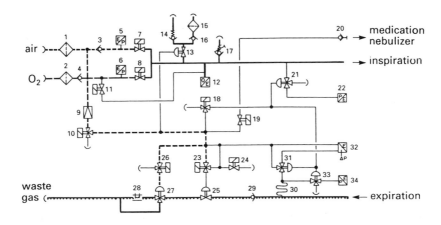

Fig. 16.14

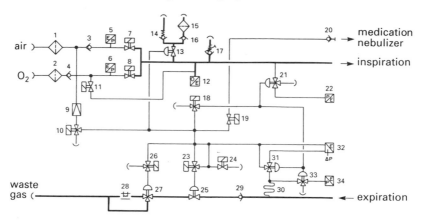

Fig. 16.15

Pressure measurement

Respiratory pathway pressure during *inspiration* is measured via bacterial trap 30 and pneumatic valve 33 at the relative pressure sensor (gauge) 34. Respiratory pathway pressure during *expiration* is measured via pneumatic valve 21 at the relative pressure sensor 22.

Differential pressure during spontaneous breathing – as a measure of the volume requirement of the patient – is measured via bacterial trap 30 and pneumatic valve 31 at the differential pressure sensor 32, whose pressure difference is acting upon the PEEP control valve 24.

Zero balance of the relative pressure sensors 22 and 34 is automatically performed by the equipment through solenoid valve 18 and pneumatic valves 21, 31 and 33, respectively. Relative pressure sensors 22 and 34 are temporarily connected to the outside air, and both measurement connections of differential pressure sensor 32 are linked to each other.

Flow measurement

The flow measurement, from which the volume determination is obtained, is performed by flow sensor 28 in the expiration line. For zero balance, pneumatic valve 27 switches the expiratory gas flow to bypass, rendering the flow sensor 28 temporarily without flow (= zero flow).

Medication atomization

Solenoid valve 19 admits a dosed air pressure flow during the inspiratory phase which is conducted to the nebulizer through gas line exit 20.

Equipment care

Technical maintenance of respirators must be performed **exclusively by the manufacturer's specially trained service technicians**. A respirator is life-saving equipment, so the life of a patient would be endangered if it were to fail at a critical moment. It is strongly recommended that a service contract be taken out with the manufacturer. **The nursing staff is, however, obliged to ensure that servicing is performed according to schedule.**

Routine equipment care by the nursing staff is limited to cleaning and disinfection. New equipment is of course delivered clean and neatly packed, but it is not sterile. Before use it has to be cleaned and disinfected just like equipment which had been used.

After *every* application, respirators must be disassembled and the hose systems must be washed in a detergent followed by thorough rinsing. For sterilization the equipment must be wrapped. Ethylene oxide sterilization is the most suitable method. The instructions of the manufacturer of the disinfectant must be followed carefully.

If plastic parts are sterilized, ethylene oxide is easily absorbed. Ethylene oxide residues can be very toxic if the aeration times are not exactly maintained. Insufficient aeration of the equipment and its accessories will cause severe damage to the lungs of the patient. If an automatic aerator is used, the aeration instructions of the manufacturer must be strictly followed. If no automatic aerator is used, the equipment must stand idle for at least 7 days before it and all its accessories can be used again on a patient.

Liquid ethylene oxide must not come into contact with plastic parts since they will be damaged.

Respirator accessories must not be touched with bare hands after complete decontamination in order to avoid any recontamination.

Daily safety check

Bird Mark series respirators

Since, as a rule, Bird respirators are used together with a Bird oxygen mixer, the user should first check the safety of this equipment. In order to do so, the plug connections for oxygen and air have each to be removed individually from the central supply line or the gas bottles, and the gas shortage alarm must go off loud and clear. The required gas pressure of 3.5 bar of both gas lines can be measured only with special measurement equipment, and should be done at regular time intervals by the hospital plant engineering department.

Assurance of correctly delivered oxygen concentration can only be obtained by continuous measurement using an oxygen monitor. This equipment should have an adjustable upper and lower limit alarm system.

(1)   Turn the equipment on, i.e. open the on/off valve on equipment having a mixing valve. On equipment that has a mixer, the reservoir bag should now inflate slightly.
(2)   Set the flow adjuster to 15 (arrow marking).
(3)   Adjust the pressure limiter to 20, which means about 20 cm water column.
(4)   Set the sensitivity lever to number 2 (arrow marking), which means about 2 cm water column.
(5)   On equipment with an air mix lever, pull this lever out and secure with catch.
(6)   Close the expiration valve by turning it to the right (clockwise).
(7)   Connect all hoses to the equipment.
(8)   To the patient side of the hoses, connect a test lung that has a capacity of about 1.5 litres. A simulated inspiration is triggered by a short push on the red bar at the sensitivity adjuster. If the system is airtight, a pressure of about 20 cm water column will now build up within the hose system and the test lung. This permits testing of the airtightness of the system. If tightness has been accomplished, the machine should now work steadily as soon as the expiration valve is opened. Make sure that during expiration the pressure indication at the manometer returns fully to zero before the next inspiration is triggered.

The desired respiration frequency cannot be tested using the test lung. For this the patient has to be connected to the respirator, and the frequency has to be controlled using a watch and a spirometer. The flow adjustment influences the inspiration time; the expiration time adjuster influences the expiration time.

Draeger Evita intensive care ventilator

An automated self-test is built into the equipment. However, the airtightness of the hose system must be tested according to the instruction manual.

Application hints

- Before every use, check equipment and accessories for visible faults.
- Always follow the manufacturer's instruction manual carefully. Since respirators frequently have to be applied very quickly, the user must be fully familiar with handling this kind of equipment.
- The components of the equipment must be assembled completely and must be functionally correct.
- Fill respiration gas humidifier with *distilled* water only and close tightly.
- Check that the equipment is functioning properly according to the instructions of the manufacturer.
- Pay particular attention to the airtightness of the complete system.
- Check proper function of all alarm systems periodically.
- Check all equipment settings, selection of the proper respiration pattern, and gas mixture composition. Only the physician decides the parameters to be used. They must never be altered without his express permission. In case of doubt call the physician.
- If possible, connect the respirator to the central monitoring system or to the nurses' call system.
- Exchange and disinfect the hose system after every patient, and at least after 24 hours of use.
- Respirator and all accessories must be cleaned and disinfected after every use, and at least after one week of use.
- Never place gas bottles near heaters or in the sun, and secure them against overturning.
- Open gas bottle valves only by hand and slowly; keep them free of oil and grease.
- Pay careful attention to the contents level of the gas bottles and keep replacement bottles at hand!
- **Patients connected to respirators must be under constant observation!**
- If the respirator is electrically driven, take care in case of power failures. Obtain information early enough about what to do in case of power failures.

Hazards

- Formation of diffuse atelectases in the event of alternate respiration (PNPB).
- Arterial oxygen pressure falls at an increasing rate as a result of

venous admixtures caused by the fact that certain areas of the lung receive less oxygen.

- Increase of afterload of the right-hand side of the heart caused by an increase in the resistance within the lung circulatory system, particularly if respiration with PEEP causes over-inflation of the alveolar space.
- 'Bronchotrauma'.
- Air trapping during the expiratory phase caused by negative pressure during intermittent over-pressure respiration if the alveoli cannot be totally ventilated owing to the collapse of the terminal bronchioli as a result of suction.
- Damage during respiration caused by the relatively frequently seen irritability of the cardiac circulatory system.
- Generalized oedema (Anasarca) during long-term artificial respiration.
- Interstitial oedema within the lungs.
- Infections within the respiratory pathways and formation of bronchopneumonias caused by inadequate hygiene.
- Toxic damage to the lungs caused by insufficient aeration of respirator and accessories after ethylene oxide sterilization.
- Obstructed gas flow caused by constrictions within the tube system (for instance by bending of the hoses); obstructions due to mucus or accumulation of condensation water.
- Faulty switch-over of the respirator to expiration, for instance due to turbulence within the bronchial system.
- Insufficient respiratory gas caused by leaks within the system, loosening of a respiration hose, faulty connection of the supply hoses to the respirator, incorrect assembly of the equipment, use of incompatible accessories, empty gas bottles, etc.
- Too high respiration pressure due to faulty equipment settings or a defect in the safety valve.
- Drying out of the respiratory pathways due to lack of water in the respiration gas humidifier; failure of the heater of the respiration gas humidifier, etc.
- Failure of the respirator or of parts of it due to damage within the electrical system of the equipment, or due to power failure.

General remarks

The German government's project group, 'Research and Development for Health Care', is developing a testing automat for respirators. This tests a multitude of pneumatic, electrical and electronic functions of electronically controlled respirators, and is being used by industry for safety testing. During its development, its use as a safety tester in hospitals as well as a demonstration and training device for medical staff has been considered. Information regarding this machine can be obtained from the 'Deutsche Forschungs- und Versuchsanstalt für Luft- und Raumfahrt (DFVLR)', Projektträgerschaften für Arbeit, Umwelt and Gesundheit, Südstrasse 125, D-5300 Bonn 2.

Further reading

Anonymous (1989) MT kurz und interessant, *MT Medizin-Technik* **1**, 3.

Bayerisches Staatsministerium für Arbeit and Sozialordnung (1986) *Sichere Technik in der Medizin*, 2nd edn, pp. 42–45.

Beneken, J.E. and Van der Aa, J.J. (1989) Alarms and their limits in monitoring, *J. Clin. Mon.* **5** (3), 205–210.

Bourke, A.E., Snowdon, S.L. and Ryan, T.D. (1987) Failure of a ventilator alarm to detect patient disconnection, *J. Med. Eng. Technol.* **11** (2), 65–67.

Bovenkamp, U. and Deterling, F. (1988) Beatmungs- und Narkosegeräte, Teil 15, *MT Medizin-Technik* **5**, 186.

Bräutigam, K.H. (1982) 3. Round-Table-Gespräch Anästhesie am 4. Juli, 1981, Technische Sicherheit beim Betrieb von Narkose- und Beatmungsgeräten, *Anästhesie und Intensivmedizin* **2**, 78.

Deutsche Gesellschaft für Anästhesie und Intensivpflege (1979) Empfehlungen der DGAI zur Sicherheit medizinisch-technischer Geräte beim Einsatz in der Anästhesiologie, *Anästhesiologie und Intensivmedizin*, 303.

Fahey, P.J. (1990) Respirator care, ventilators, resuscitators, *Medical Electronics* **21** (1), 154–156.

Fahey, P.J. (1993) Respirator care, ventilators, resuscitators, *Medical Electronics* **24** (1), 127–129.

Frankenberger, H., Bender, H.J., Ryll, C. and van Ackern, K. (1992) Alarmverhalten verschiedener Beatmungsgeräte beim Auftreten klinisch relevanter Störfälle, *MT Medizin Technik* **112** (3), 90–101.

Guyton, A.C. (1961) *Medical Physiology*, W.B. Saunders Co., Philadelphia.

Hahn, C. and Hesse, F.W. (1991) Action generation in system control: theoretical considerations and empirical findings, Progress Report 4PR 4.1 RHK ESPRIT BRA 3219 KAUDYTE, Institute for Psychology, Georg-August Universität Göttingen, Germany.

Hahn, C., Hesse, F.W. and Cornelius, K. (1993) Handhabung von Beatmungsgeräten in der Intensivpflege, *MT Medizin Technik* **113** (4), 130–133.

Kerr, J.A. (1985) Warning devices, *Brit. J. Anaesth.* **57**, 696–708.

Knaack-Steinegger, R. and Thomson, D.A. (1989) The measurement of expiratory oxygen as disconnection alarm, *Anesthesiology* **44** (12), 994–995.

Kreysch, W. (1984) *Grundlagen der Beatmung*, Verlag TÜV, Rheinland.

Lawin, P. (1971) *Praxis der Intensivbehandlung*, p. 261 ff, G. Thieme Verlag, Stuttgart.

McEven, J.A., Small, C.F. and Jenkins, L.C. (1988) Detection of interruptions in the breathing gas of ventilated anaesthetized patients, *Canad. J. Anaesth.* **35** (6), 549–561.

Ministerium für Arbeit und Soziales des Landes Nordrhein Westfalen (1987) *Studie zur Verbesserung der Sicherheit von Beatmungs- und Narkosegeräten.*

Myerson, K.R., Ilsley, A.H. and Runciman, W.B. (1986) An evaluation of ventilator monitoring alarms, *Anaesth. Intensive Care* **14** (2), 174–185.

Pryn, S.J. and Crosse, M.M. (1989) Ventilator disconnection alarm failures. The role of ventilator and breathing system accessories, *Anesthesia* **44** (12), 978–981.

Quinn, M.L. (1989) Semipractible alarms: a parable, *J. Clin. Mon.* **5** (3), 196–200.

Rathgeber, J. (1987) Beatmung, in Feilbot *et al.*: *Praktische Gerätetechnik*, Verlag Medizinische Kongress-Organisation, Nürnberg.

Chapter 17
Defibrillators

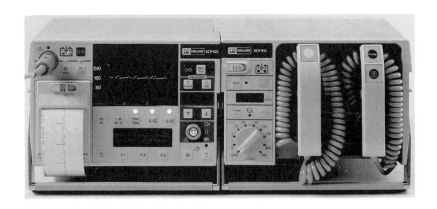

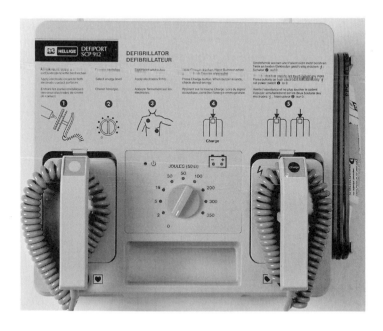

Examples of defibrillators.

Principle of operation

Life-threatening arrhythmias such as cardiac fibrillation, cardiac flutter, tachycardias and the like can be interrupted very efficiently by defibrillation. The defibrillator applies an adjustable electrical pulse directly to the heart (Fig. 17.1).

A modern defibrillator consists of four main components:

- the *electrical supply*, which is obtained either from the electrical distribution system or from a battery;
- the *electrical charging circuit*, which charges the energy storage system, usually a condenser (capacitor);
- the *energy storage capacitor*, which can be charged to up to 5000 volts; and
- the *discharge circuit* through which the defibrillation pulse is delivered and which influences its shape. In the case of external defibrillation, energies of about 20 to 360 joules (joule is the unit of energy, 1 Joule = 0.2390 calories) are delivered, depending upon the body weight of the patient. This means 1100–3000 volts at a current of 22 to 60 amperes and a pulse duration of 3 to 8 milliseconds.

Electrical defibrillation is the most important measure in cases of cardiac fibrillation. The earlier defibrillation is started, the more successful it will be. The defibrillation pulse causes depolarization of all

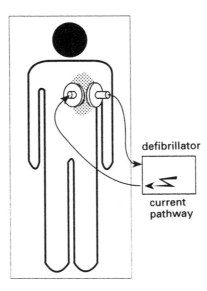

Fig. 17.1   Current pathway of the defibrillating pulse.

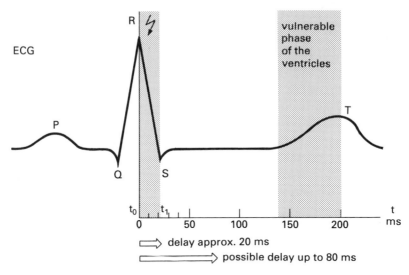

Fig. 17.2 Electrical trigger point at cardioversion.

cardiac muscle fibres which are capable of being stimulated, i.e. which are not yet within the absolute refractory phase. Since fibrillating fibres have a greatly shortened refractory phase, the pulse will accomplish simultaneous depolarization of the entire myocardium as well as of the pulse transmitting system. The heart is as it were electrically switched to zero. After this coordination, the sino-atrial node can again take over its leading role as the pacemaker.

In electrical interruption of atrial arrhythmias, the electrical pulse should never fall into the vulnerable phase since this could trigger ventricular flutter or fibrillation. In this case, a defibrillator coupled with an ECG is used which will trigger the pulse by synchronization with the R-wave of the ECG. This kind of defibrillation is also called cardioversion (Fig. 17.2).

Since the R–T interval is on average 300 400 ms and even at tachycardia under influence of digitalis never goes below 200 ms, the safety of synchronization (cardioversion) is quite adequate. Even in the event of bundle branch blocks or extra-systoles, 20 ms after the R-wave no fibrillation can be triggered.

However, successful defibrillation requires a constant, sufficient oxygen supply for the patient.

Equipment care

Although application of the defibrillator is, as a rule, reserved for the physician, **it is the responsibility of the nurse to take care that the defibrillator is always immediately ready for use if needed**. In order to ensure this, the following rules must be observed:

- Patient cables and electrodes should never get entangled. Make sure that one grip on the electrodes gets them and the cables immediately separate from each other out of the housing of the equipment. **Tangled-up patient cables mean loss of valuable treatment time!**
- Cables and electrodes must always be clean, particularly of electrode gel residues. If this is not the case, the defibrillating physician may get part of the defibrillation shock himself when triggering the defibrillator.
- Battery-operation defibrillators must always have a completely charged battery. Whether used or not, connect the defibrillator once every week to the electrical power line for 24 hours in order to recharge the battery. **After every use of the defibrillator, always recharge the battery fully again**.
- The most important part of the defibrillator is its energy storage capacitor. As with most electronic components, current must flow through it from time to time or it will deteriorate. You should switch on your defibrillator at least every 4 weeks, charge it up to maximum load (360 Joules), and subsequently discharge it again by resetting the charge adjustment to zero in order to ensure that the capacitor is and remains in good condition.
- Ensure that the defibrillator is inspected for safety regularly and according to regulations. Should any faults or irregularities be found, have the equipment *immediately* maintained and/or repaired.

Daily safety check

As has already been mentioned, there will be little time for testing the defibrillator if it is needed. It is therefore important to perform such testing at regular intervals, at least once a week. In order to avoid any problems in the event of an accident, this test should be documented by the person performing it.

The test should be carried out by the nurse as follows:

(1) Switch the defibrillator on and set the energy adjuster to 360 Joules.
(2) Push the charge button. The full charge must be obtained within 15 seconds.

(3) For battery-operated defibrillators, five full charges must be possible within 15 seconds each. Thereafter, another two full charges must be possible, within a little more time. **Should this not be possible, the defibrillator must be sent for inspection and repair at once!**

(4) Full discharge (discharge button or resetting of energy adjuster) must not take longer than 10 seconds.

Application hints

Prepare the defibrillator for the physician by evenly distributing a *thin* layer of electrode gel. Too much electrode gel may cause the physician to come into contact with it and hence obtain part of the electrical shock himself. In addition, too much gel may form a conductive bridge between the electrodes on the skin of the patient so that part of the defibrillator shock remains at the skin surface and hence does not reach the heart. Too little electrode gel may cause severe burns on the skin of the patient.

Figure 17.3 shows the defibrillator energy normally required according to the patient's body weight. As a rule, one begins using 200 joules and increases gradually as required up to 360 joules (more is legally not permissible). For adult patients adjust the defibrillator first to 200 joules unless the physician requests otherwise.

If the physician orders a change of defibrillation energy, always

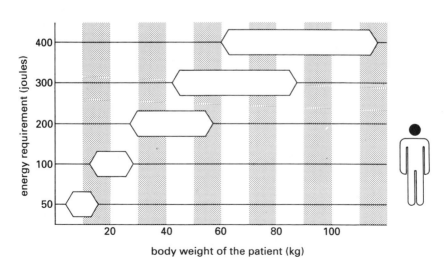

Fig. 17.3 Average necessary defibrillation energy according to body weight of the patient.

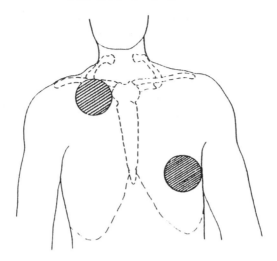

Fig. 17.4   Electrode placement for anterior–anterior defibrillation.

discharge the defibrillator first (turn adjuster back to zero and wait until discharge is indicated), and subsequently, adjust to the new energy as ordered and charge up.

Take care that the patient is not in contact with any electrically conductive parts (bed rail, etc.) and that there are no sharp corners nearby on which the patient (or the physician) could get hurt.

The body of the patient must be dry. Humidity (sweat) is electrically conductive, so in its presence a conductive bridge between the electrodes could result through which part of the defibrillation pulse could be deviated. This means loss of energy to the heart.

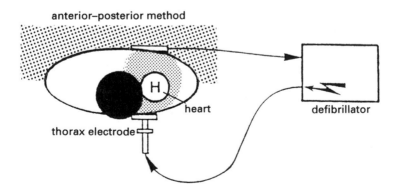

Fig. 17.5   Electrode placement for anterior–posterior defibrillation (cardioversion).

Normally, the anterior–anterior method is applied, i.e. both electrodes are placed on the chest of the patient as shown in Fig. 17.4.

For cardioversion, the anterior-posterior method is usually preferred, i.e. one electrode to the chest, the other one to the back of the patient (Fig. 17.5).

Never touch any metal parts in the surroundings of the patient (bed rail, etc.). If the patient should by chance touch these, you will get part of the defibrillation pulse yourself!

The defibrillation pulse should if possible be triggered during expiration of the patient since in this case the distance from the skin surface and hence from the electrode to the heart is shorter. During inspiration there is a lot of air between electrode and heart, and air is not a good electrical conductor.

Hazards

For the user

- Electrical shock by contact with the electrode or other parts which may possibly carry electricity.
- Injury caused by sharp corners if the user gets part of the electrical shock and pulls back sharply.

For the patient

- Too high defibrillation energy may cause burns or internal injury.
- Too low defibrillation energy causes loss of valuable therapy time which may be fatal for the patient.
- An implanted cardiac pacemaker might be damaged by the defibrillation pulse and become useless. Always have a replacement (external) pacemaker ready for emergencies.
- Other equipment connected to the patient (monitors, ECG, etc.) may be damaged by the defibrillation shock and fail. Leave only equipment connected to the patient during defibrillation which is defibrillator proof (they carry the sign ⊣♥⊢).
- Think also of the possibility of 'secondary accidents', for instance patients making violent motions caused by fright triggered by the defibrillation shock, striking against sharp corners and hurts themselves. Such accidents are not as rare as one might like to believe.

General remarks

Defibrillators are life-saving equipment. They must therefore be maintained regularly and be given regular safety inspections.

Further reading

Ahnefeld, F.W. *et al.* (1991) *Richtlinien für Wiederbelebung und Notfallversorgung*, Deutscher Ärzteverlag, Cologne.

Anonymous (1986) Standards and guidelines for cardiopulmonary resuscitation (CPR) and emergency cardiac care (ECC), *J.A.M.A.* **255**, 2905, 2946.

Anonymous (1989) Defibrillators, *Medical Electronics* **20** (5), 153–154.

Bayerisches Staatministerium für Arbeit und Sozialordnung (1986) *Sichere Technik in der Medizin*, 2nd edn, pp. 40–42.

DIN-VDE 0753, Teil 3 (1983) Anwendungsregeln für Defibrillatoren.

Dubin, D.B. (1981) *Schnellinterpretation des EKG*, Springer Verlag, Berlin.

Knapp, H.P. (1988) Defibrillatoren, Technik und Umgang, *Intensivbehandlung* **13** (3).

Kresse, H. (1982) *Kompendium der Elektromedizin*, Siemens AG, Erlangen.

Lindner, K.H., Ahnefeld, F.W., Lotz, P. and Rossi, P. (1986) Cardiopulmonale reanimation, Ambu Internatl, Copenhagen.

Lüderitz, B. (1984) *Therapie der Herzrhythmusstörungen*, Springer Verlag, Berlin.

Merz, U. (1989) *Einführung in die Interpretation des EKG*, Elektrotherapie, Hellige, Freiburg.

Schlepper, M. and Issen, B. (1983) *Kardiale Rhythmusstörungen*, Springer Verlag, Berlin.

Thorspecken, R. and Hassenslein, P. (1975) *Rhythmusstörungen des Herzens*, G. Thieme Verlag, Stuttgart.

Chapter 18
Haemodialysis Equipment

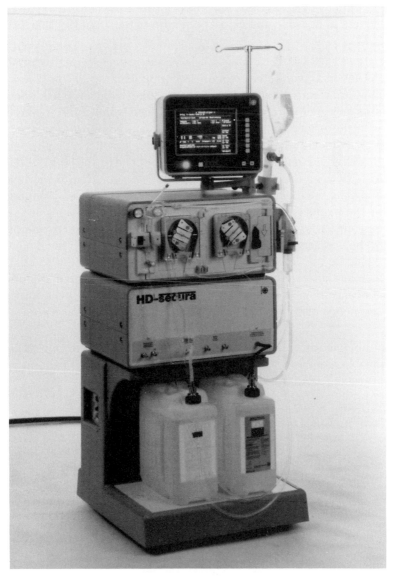

Typical haemodialysis machine.

Principle of operation

Haemodialysis is the purification of blood within an artificial kidney (dialysator) by transport of matter through a membrane into the cleansing solution (dialysation liquid). This kind of treatment becomes necessary in the event of temporary failure of kidney function (acute nephroparalysis) or in continuous chronic kidney failure (terminal kidney insufficiency). It is the purpose of this treatment to replace, as effectively as possible, the natural function of the kidneys. Thus its role is:

- to decontaminate the blood. Decontamination of the blood is important since, during metabolism, toxic final products such as urea, uric acid and creatinine are produced which must be excreted with the urine. If these substances remain within the body of the patient, self-intoxication will occur which will be finally lethal. However, not only do toxic products produced by the body itself lead to toxicity; a lot of other toxic substances admitted to the human body, e.g. medicines, caffeine, nicotine, etc., must also be excreted by the kidneys.
- to maintain liquid balance. If liquids are not excreted, an overflooding of the body causing oedema formation, particularly within the lungs, would be the consequence.
- to maintain electrolyte balance. Alterations within the electrolyte concentrations would cause dysfunctions within the muscular cells and hence also possible dysfunctions of the cardiac activities.

In the dialysator, liquids and matter are transported through a semipermeable membrane. The transport is based on the physical principles of diffusion, ultrafiltration and osmosis.

Diffusion (Fig. 18.1)

If there are two solutions of different concentration within one container separated by a membrane which is permeable to the matter dissolved in the solution, migration of the dissolved matter through the membrane will take place until equalization of the concentration is accomplished. The movement is always from the higher to the lower concentration. The speed depends upon:

- the degree of difference in concentration,
- the thickness of the membrane,

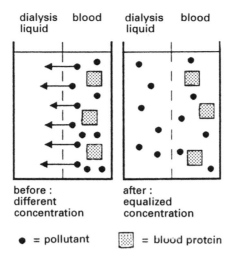

before :
different
concentration

after :
equalized
concentration

● = pollutant   ▦ = blood protein

Fig. 18.1 Principle of diffusion.

- the characteristics of the pores (size and condition),
- the area of the membrane,
- the temperature of the solutions (which is of little importance in haemodialysis since the temperature of the dialysation liquid and the body temperature of the patient, and hence also of the blood, must be approximately the same),
- the membrane contact time of the matter (since, in haemodialysis, blood and dialysation liquid pass each other flowing in different directions).

Since the concentration of pollutants in the blood decreases on its way through the dialysator whereas saturation of pollutants increases within the dialysation liquid, both liquids are conducted to flow in opposite directions (following the counter-flow principle). This ensures that, at every point on the membrane, there will be an approximately equal drop in concentration.

Ultrafiltration (Fig. 18.2)

If, within a container in which two liquids are separated by a permeable membrane, a positive pressure (hyperpressure) is built up on one side and a negative pressure (suction) is built up on the other side, all matter dissolved in the solution which can penetrate the membrane will be transported to the part of the container having the lower pressure. The

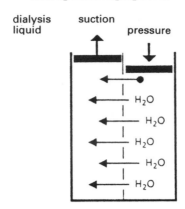

Fig. 18.2   Principle of ultrafiltration.

amount of matter transported through the membrane (the ultrafiltration capacity) depends upon:

- the difference in pressure at the membrane (TMP = transmembranous pressure),
- the porous density,
- the properties of the membrane (size of the pores, condition of the pores, thickness of the membrane).

The ultrafiltration capacity of a dialysator is indicated by the manufacturer using the ultrafiltration factor (k-factor).

During haemodialysis, dissolved matter will also be transported together with the solvent during ultrafiltration because of the structure of the membrane. This flow causes, in addition, transport of matter convectively.

Osmosis (Fig. 18.3)

The withdrawal of liquid can also be caused by osmosis. If there are two liquids of different concentrations within a container, separated from each other by a membrane that is permeable for the liquids, transport of liquid through the membrane will also happen without any hydrostatic pressure. In this case the liquid that has the higher concentration will try to reduce its concentration until equilibrium of both concentrations is accomplished.

For removal of water during dialysis, glucose is added to the dialysation liquid until its concentration is higher than that in the blood. Because of their size, the glucose molecules cannot penetrate through

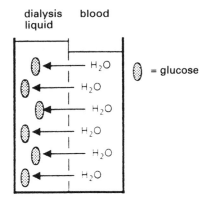

Fig. 18.3 Principle of osmosis.

the membrane. Hence, water molecules move from the blood to the dialysation liquid to produce an equilibrium there.

This method is today of only secondary importance in haemodialysis because of the infection hazard involved. However, it is still used in peritoneal dialysis.

Peritoneal dialysis is a therapy method in which exchange of matter is performed within the coeliac space through the peritoneum (which serves here as the membrane). The risk of infection is quite high when using this method. This is because large quantities of glucose-contained dialysation solution immediately fill the coeliac space, and after completion of the exchange of matter are removed from it. Unless great care is taken, there is a serious risk of, among other hazards, peritonitis. Reasons for preferring peritoneal dialysis include:

- insufficient blood flow (small children, the elderly),
- no possibility of punctures,
- psychological considerations,
- eventual use in home dialysis since little technical expertise is necessary.

Summary

In haemodialysis, withdrawal of liquid is accomplished by ultrafiltration (hydrostatic pressure), and detoxification is accomplished by diffusion (difference in concentration) and by convective transport of matter (in ultrafiltration). To accomplish this it is necessary to let the specially prepared dialysation liquid and the blood of the patient pass each other in a controlled way.

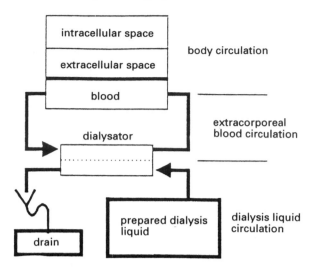

Fig. 18.4   Simplified representation of the different liquid circulations.

The different liquid circulations (Fig. 18.4)

In addition to the blood circulation within the body of the patient, we have to differentiate between the extracorporeal blood circulation and the dialysation liquid circulation.

Blood vessel access

For haemodialysis a sufficiently high blood flow (around 200–300 ml/min) is necessary. In order to be able to extract such an amount of blood from the patient, an artery that is not easily accessible (for instance the arteria radialis) would have to be punctured. Since it would not be

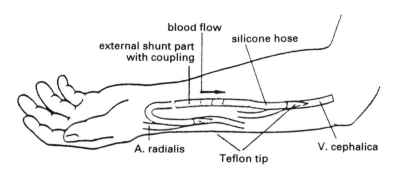

Fig. 18.5   Scribner shunt.

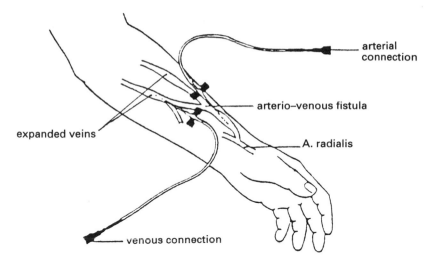

arterial
connection

arterio–venous fistula

expanded veins

A. radialis

venous connection

Fig. 18.6 Cimino fistula.

possible to do this three times weekly over many years, an artificial puncturing point has to be created. Either a point of access located outside the body is surgically provided (a Scribner shunt, Fig. 18.5), or an arterio-venous connection located directly under the skin (a Cimino fistula, Fig. 18.6) is prepared. Today the Cimino fistula is generally used. For the Scribner shunt, the connection to the extracorporeal circulation is provided by means of couplings of the hoses. For the Cimino fistula, punctures through the skin into the vessel are necessary.

Extracorporeal circulation (Fig. 18.7)

The extracorporeal circulation brings the contaminated blood to be dialysed from the patient to the dialysator and the cleaned blood from the dialysator back to the patient. This extracorporeal circulation consists mainly of special blood-conducting hoses, the puncture cannula, and the dialysator. For reasons of hygiene, all these parts are provided as disposable accessories.

In order to maintain a sufficient and even flow of blood, the blood is pumped from the patient into the extracorporeal circulation by means of a *blood pump*. Maximal flow of blood is limited by the amount of blood available at the puncture site of the patient.

Since blood coagulates as soon as it leaves the natural surroundings of the blood vessel and comes into contact with the rough plastic surface of the hoses and the dialysator, an anticoagulant, for instance heparin, has to be added to it. The heparin doses may be added during the entire

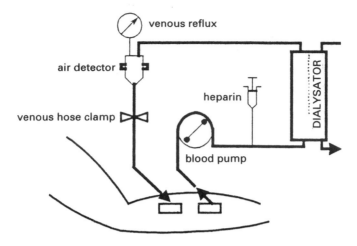

Fig. 18.7   Simplified representation of the extracorporeal blood circulation.

dialysis treatment (around 4–5 hours) continuously by means of an inbuilt infusion pump, or manually at given time intervals (intermittently).

The blood flows through the dialysator and reaches an enlargement in the blood conducting hose, the *venous bubble trap*. Here, any air bubbles that may have entered the blood are trapped. This might be cause by leaky hoses or hose connections, or by carelessness in connecting the patient to the machine. Penetration of air into the blood circulatory system of the patient, either as a single air bubble or as blood foam, is a considerable hazard and hence must be avoided.

Air bubbles or blood foam are recognized by the *air detector* within the venous bubble trap. This surveillance system interrupts the blood flow to the patient by closing the *venous hose clamp* if the air or foam quantities can no longer be absorbed by the bubble trap. This will also stop the blood pump.

To the venous bubble trap is connected a pressure shunt which monitors the *venous back-flow pressure*. The venous back-flow pressure must not be confused with the blood pressure of the patient. It is a technical measurement value which results from the flow conditions within the hose system and the venous connection to the patient. This pressure control permits recognition of leakages within the extracorporeal circulation as well as hindrances to the blood flow caused by bends or obstructions of the hose, or of the venous cannula by blood clots.

Dialysation liquid circulation (Fig. 18.8)

Within the dialysation liquid circulation, the cleansing liquid is prepared in such a way that matter and liquid are extracted from the blood of the patient in a controlled way. Since drinking water contains many substances which may cause complications during dialysis, it must be upgraded to *pure water* by suitable procedures (reverse osmosis, desalination, etc.).

To avoid cooling down the blood within the extracorporeal circulation, the pure water is warmed to body temperature by a heater. The selectable temperature range is, as a rule, set at 35– 40°C. It is necessary to ensure, by means of a protective system, that no dialysation liquid with a temperature greater than 41°C can enter the dialysator since any liquid with a temperature of 42.6°C or more will damage the blood by haemolysis and protein denaturization.

Water contains dissolved gas which is released as bubbles during warming and at under-pressure. Since, for the purpose of ultrafiltration, an underpressure of 400 to 500 mmHg is produced within the dialysator, gas bubbles may be formed which would reduce the effective membrane surface and hence also reduce the efficiency of the treatment. They might also penetrate through the membrane into the blood where they could produced blood foam. In order to avoid this, the water is first degassed, i.e. freed from the dissolved gas by means of under-pressure.

The degassed and warmed water is prepared within a mixing system with a concentrate (concentrated salt solution having an exactly defined

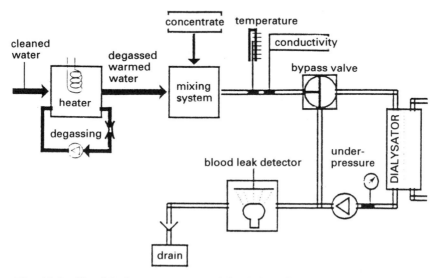

Fig. 18.8 Simplified representation of the dialysis liquid circulation.

composition) in a predetermined proportion (usually 34:1) to become the required dialysation liquid. The composition of the dialysation liquid corresponds basically to the composition of the blood and has to be such that:

- substances which have to be removed from the blood are present at low concentration or not at all,
- substances which have to be delivered to the blood are present at higher concentration,
- substances of which no exchange is intended are present at a concentration equal to that within the blood.

After the mixing process, temperature and conductance of the dialysation liquid are measured. They are indicated on a meter, and hence can be monitored throughout the entire dialysis treatment time. The electrical conductance of the solution permits an indirect conclusion to be made about its composition, provided the composition of the concentrate used is known.

If one of the control systems recognizes any fault within the dialysation liquid circulation, the faulty liquid is conducted through the bypass valve away from the dialysator (position shown in Fig. 18.8). This makes this valve one of the most important safety features in addition to the sensors.

For dialysis, the bypass valve is switched to the pass position and the liquid flows through the dialysator. Here, the exchange of matter and water removal take place.

For controlled ultrafiltration a hydrostatic pressure has to be built up by means of an under-pressure pump. A measurement system controls the pressure build-up because, in the event of too high an under-pressure, too much is ultrafiltrated and the dialysator membrane might be destroyed. During normal pressure conditions it is also possible that the membrane might be damaged (rupture). In this case, in addition to the substances to be dialysed, solid blood constituents such as white and red blood cells pass into the dialysation liquid. In these circumstances the blood leak detector recognizes the blood within the dialysation liquid and switches the equipment to the 'safe condition', i.e. the bypass valve conducts the dialysation liquid away from the dialysator.

After the dialysation liquid has passed the blood leak detector it is conducted, inclusive of the ultrafiltrate, into the drain.

Equipment care

In order to protect the patient and the user from infections, the following procedure must be carried out after **every** use of the equipment.

- Clean the housing of the dialysis equipment of blood and other forms of contamination and disinfect it with a disinfectant approved by the manufacturer. Take care that no solution can enter into the equipment.
- Clean and disinfect the dialysation liquid circulation system according to the manufacturer's instructions. Both chemical and heat disinfection are possible. Subsequently, the equipment must be cooled down and thoroughly rinsed in order to remove all residual chemical disinfectant.
- It is important to make sure that the equipment cannot by accident be used for therapy during the disinfection process (for instance by locking it away). The blood of the patient would be severely damaged by heat or disinfectants.
- The blood hose system, the dialysator and the cannula are disposable equipment. Special care must be taken to ensure that they are disposed of safely (infectious material may be present).

Daily safety check

Before every use the user must check all alarms and safety provisions. To do this, all alarm limits are deliberately overburdened and the triggering of the alarm as well as any consequent effects on the equipment (bypass valve, hose closing clamp, stopping of blood pump, etc.) are checked.

Since this is a very elaborate procedure which is probably not within the technical capability of every user, the provision of an automatic test unit is strongly recommended. A safety check using such equipment ensures reliable and safe treatment of the patient.

In addition it is important to ensure that the equipment is properly assembled and that all parts are correctly and completely connected. A visual check must also be made that the equipment has no visible external damage (a broken line cord or connector, etc.).

Application hints

Before using the equipment, check for the following:

- Are all the connections of the equipment correctly attached?
- Has the equipment been correctly cleaned and sterilized?
- Is the equipment free of residues of the disinfectant?

- Is the concentrate mixture correct according to the doctor's prescription?
- Is the quantity of concentrate sufficient for the treatment?
- Is the concentrate supply line correctly connected?
- Are the prescribed values for temperature and concentration (conductance) properly adjusted?
- Are the blood hose systems and the dialysator being used suitable and sterile?
- Is the blood hose system correctly connected, flushed and free of air?
- Are all operative values of the equipment correctly adjusted?
- Are all critical alarm values properly selected?
- Does the indicated value for conductance and for temperature correspond to the prescribed values?
- Is the dialysator free of air?
- Is the flow direction of the dialysation liquid correct?
- Are any leaks recognizable within the dialysator and the blood hose system?
- Is sufficient heparin available for the treatment?

The safety of the patient is assured only if all safety devices have been tested before every use, and if they are not bypassed during treatment.

A comfortable position for the patient must be provided. During treatment, a nurse must be permanently within the room in order to take immediate action in the event of any malfunction.

Hazards

For the user

- The risk of infections, particularly in the case of patients who have infectious diseases such as hepatitis, AIDS, etc.
- The possibility of injury when handling the cannulas and during insertion of the hoses into the pump systems.
- Hazard of electrical shock caused by wet or humid electrical connections or faulty cables or connectors.
- Injury of skin or eyes by solutions or vapour of aggressive disinfectants or detergents.

For the patient

- Hazard of embolism caused by incorrect or insufficient air removal from hose systems or by air contained within a defective air trap.

- Hazard of thrombosis, for instance where the dose of anticoagulants is insufficient.
- Too much mechanical stress, caused, for instance, by the blood pump.
- Faulty preparation of the dialysation liquid.
- Acute incompatibility reactions with applied materials or chemical substances adhering to them.
- Bleeding caused by faulty alteration of the blood coagulation (hyperheparinization).
- Blood losses caused by unintentional removal of the cannula, detachment of hose connections, or rupture of the membrane within the dialysator (blood leakage).
- Failure of control systems.
- Removal of too much liquid from the blood.
- Wrong temperature of the dialysation liquid.
- Residual disinfectant within the dialysation liquid circulation.
- Faulty application of the dialysis equipment.
- Wrong position of the puncture cannula.
- Too strong or insufficient ultrafiltration.
- Calculation errors.
- Infections.
- Electrical or mechanical hazards caused by defective dialysis equipment.

Special risks of peritoneal dialysis

- Injuries caused by the catheter.
- Non-sterile equipment and conditions.
- Application of too high or too low quantities of rinsing liquid.
- The rinsing liquid present within the coelium for the wrong length of time.
- Application during peritonitis is contraindicated.

General remarks

Haemodialysis equipment must be applied only within rooms especially provided for this purpose.

It is strongly recommended that service contracts be taken out with the equipment manufacturer.

Further reading

Bayerisches Staatsministerium für Arbeit und Sozialordnung (1980) *Sichere Technik in der Medizin,* 2nd edn, pp. 49–53.

Böckmann, R-D. (1985) *Dialysegeräte, Grundlagen,* Verlag TÜV Rheinland, Cologne.

Brescia, M.J., Cimino, J.E., Appel, K. and Huntrich, B.J. (1966) Chronic hemodialysis using venipunture and surgically created arterio-venous fistula, *New Engl. J. Med.* **275**, 2089.

DIN VDE 0750, Teil 206 (1986) Haemodialysegeräte; besondere Festlegung für die Sicherheit.

DIN VDE 0753, Teil 4 (1986) Anwendungsregeln für Haemodialysegeräte.

Franz, H.E. (1984) *Dialysebehandlung,* G. Thieme Verlag, Stuttgart.

Friedman, E.A. and Mellins, J. (1964) Metastatic calcification and pseudogout complicating chronic dialysis, *Proc. Working Conf. Chron. Dial.* **130**.

Ministerium für Arbeit, Gesundheit und Soziales des Landes Nordrhein-Westfalen (1989) Studie zur Verbesserung der Sicherheit von Dialyseverfahren und Dialysegeräten.

Renking, E.M. (1956) The relation between dialysance, membrane, beta area, permeability, and blood flow in the artificial kidney, *Trans. Amer. Soc. artif. intern. Organs* **2**, 210.

Schreiner, G.E. (1958) Role of hemodialysis (artificial kidney) in acute poisoning, *Arch. Intern. Med.* **102**, 896.

Chapter 19
High Frequency Surgical Equipment

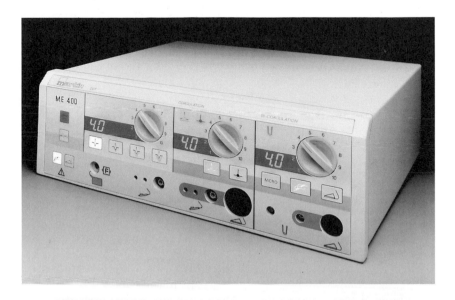

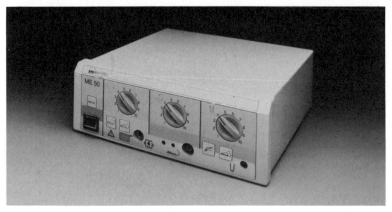

Examples of high frequency surgery machines.

Principle of operation

If electricity passes through biological tissues, the following effects can be observed:

- a thermal effect (development of heat),
- an electrolytic effect, and
- a stimulating effect.

In high frequency surgery – referred to in what follows as Hf-surgery – only the thermal effect is of important whereas the stimulating and electrolytic effects interfere and can even be dangerous; hence they are unwanted.

The thermal effect

Biological tissues are heated if electrical current passes through them. The quantity of this heating depends upon:

- the specific resistance of such tissues to electricity (in ohm/cm^2),
- the current intensity (in amperes),
- the current density, and
- the time the electricity interacts with the tissues.

The *specific resistance* of the tissue varies from case to case. Tissues consisting of dense cell membranes, partially of cells that are dying off or already dead (for instance the epidermis), have a very high electrical resistance (up to 20 000 ohms and more), whereas young tissues with a good blood supply, as are found inside the body, have quite a low electrical resistance (20 ohms and less).

The *current intensity* can be adjusted by means of a control on the Hf-surgery equipment. It must be remembered, however, that too high a current intensity might unintentionally also damage tissue surrounding the area of surgery, and that on the other hand a cutting effect can only be accomplished with a sufficiently high current intensity. The selection of the proper current intensity is hence of decisive importance.

Of fundamental importance is the *current density*. The smaller the area of current supply, the stronger is the effect of the current. The reverse also holds true: the larger the area of current supply the lower is the effect of the current (Fig. 19.1).

We can therefore summarize as follows:

High current density = high current effect
Low current density = low current effect

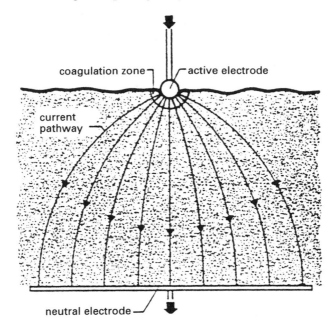

Fig. 19.1 Example of low and high current density.

The active electrode of an Hf-surgery machine, i.e. the cutting or coagulating electrode, must therefore have a high current density whereas the passive electrode which leads the electrical current away must have a low current density.

What has been said above shows clearly why it is so important that the passive electrode, also called the plate, be in complete contact with the body of the patient in order to utilize its full area and hence to reduce the current effect to almost zero. If this is not the case, many small contact 'islands' exist, distributed irregularly over the plate area. These will have a higher current density than intended, and an unwanted current effect might occur producing electrical burns.

The *interaction time* of the current with the tissue is of importance as the electrical resistance will rise owing to the destruction of cells within the tissue and hence the thermal effect will become more pronounced.

The electrolytic effect

If electrical current flows through biological tissues, it will cause movement of ions. If this current is a DC (direct current), the positively charged ions of the tissue will migrate towards the negative pole, the cathode, and the negatively charged ions will migrate towards the positive pole, the anode. In these circumstances the tissues would be damaged electrolytically by unphysiologically high ion concentrations. In order to avoid this, AC (alternating current) is used for Hf-surgery.

The stimulating effect

It has been demonstrated by experimental investigations (Quilligan 1968, von der Mosel 1971 a, b) that with increasing frequency of an AC (alternating current) from 100 Hertz upwards, the stimulating effect of electrical current decreases and disappears fully at about 150 kilohertz (Fig. 19.2). For this reason, AC at frequencies of more than 300 kilohertz is used for Hf-surgery (hence the term 'high-frequency'). **It must, however, be pointed out that, even at such high frequencies, the functioning of implanted cardiac pacemakers still can be affected**.

The Hf-surgery technique as described above, where the electrical current is conducted away from the patient by means of a plate electrode, is called the *monopolar* technique. In the *bipolar* technique, a double polar active electrode is used instead of the plate electrode; the electrical current is conducted to and from the surgery site through one of the two active electrodes (referred to as forceps or forks because of their shape) which are arranged close to each other. In this case, a plate electrode to conduct the electrical current away from the patient is not necessary. This technique is particularly suitable for smaller local surgical procedures. It has the advantage that the current will flow through only a small area of the body of the patient provided there is no contact elsewhere with any electrical connection to ground (water pipe, metallic table top, etc.). In this case, the effect on implanted cardiac pacemakers is reduced (**but not excluded!**).

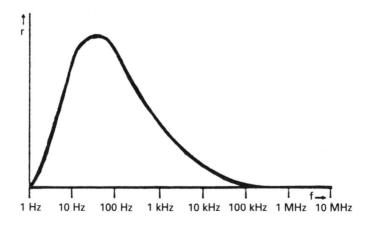

Fig. 19.2 Dependency of stimulating effect of AC on current frequency.

Equipment care

As with the defibrillator, application of Hf-surgical equipment is usually reserved for the physician, whereas preparation and (if no biomedical engineering technician is available) maintenance of the equipment are the duty of the nursing staff. To ensure perfect function and safe and hygienic application of the equipment, the following maintenance guidelines must be observed:

- Using steel wool, clean the active electrode of tissue residues before sterilization.
- Pack active electrodes, electrode handles and the cables and connectors belonging to them in cloth and sterilize in steam at up to 134°C. Thereafter, unpack them immediately from the humid cloth and dry them well. Objects with hollow spaces (e.g. electrode handles) must be thoroughly shaken out in order to remove water condensate.
- Clean the neutral electrode with the cables, connectors, and fixing straps belonging to them and rub them off with a disinfectant. They must also be completely dry before reuse.
- Clean and disinfect foot switch and generator housing only if they are very dirty, using a moist cloth only. Ensure that no liquid penetrates into them.
- **Never use any inflammable detergents to clean Hf-surgical equipment and accessories.**
- **Carefully avoid penetration of any liquids into Hf-surgical equipment and accessories.**
- **Never use hot air drying or sterilization for this kind of equipment.** This would damage plastic parts and the soldering joints of the equipment.
- After cleaning and disinfection, always check all electrical cables and connectors for damage and effective contacts. Send any damaged parts **immediately** for repair, otherwise the operating physician will be in danger of severe burns.

Daily safety check

Follow carefully the instructions of the user's manual for this test. In addition, the following must be observed carefully.

- Inspect the plate electrode.

○ *Metallic* plate electrodes must be clean and shiny. Any oxidation (dull grey staining) must be carefully removed using steel wool or sandpaper. The plates must not be bent or dented since otherwise it would not be possible to ensure complete contact with the skin of the patient.

○ Plates made of *conductive rubber* must be clean, not greasy, and not brittle. Look particularly for 'scalds' which originate from touching the active electrode on the plate while the generator is switched on in order to 'test' the proper function of the equipment by means of the spark visible in this procedure. Doing this is a serious fault since at this location the plate is consequently severely damaged.

● Check for the good condition and correct connection of all cables and connectors.
● Check that the equipment, foot switch, electrodes and all other accessories are absolutely dry.
● Switch the equipment on and check the proper functioning of all control lamps and safety provisions.
● Check that the correct electrode is in the handle (mono- or bipolar cutting electrode, or ball or flat electrode for coagulation, etc.).

Application hints

Before the equipment is used it is the duty of the nursing staff to prepare it and the patient properly. In doing so observe the following guidelines.

Patient

● Improve the electrical conductivity of the skin of the patient by cleaning it of fat and, where necessary (when there is horny skin and scars), by careful rubbing with physiological saline solution.
● Position the patient in such a way that he cannot come into contact with any electrically conductive parts (metal parts of the operating table, holding supports, wet cloth, etc.). Between patient, operating table and holding supports, an electrically insulating, dry, thick lining must be placed, which must stay dry throughout application of Hf-surgery.
● Fasten the neutral electrode securely to the body of the patient in such a way that it cannot become loose if the patient should move. Despite the necessity for good fixation, take care that no pressure is applied that could interrupt the circulation and lead to necrosis. Remove dense hair growth from the application site first.

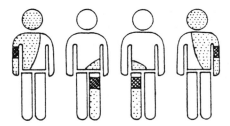

Fig. 19.3 Placement of neutral electrode depending on location of Hf-surgery.

- Do not apply the electrode directly over larger blood vessels near the skin surface.
- Keep the current pathway between active and neutral electrodes as short as possible. Figure 19.3 shows where the neutral electrode should be located for particular operating areas.
- If the patient is connected to any monitoring device during surgery (for example an ECG monitor), the neutral ECG cable (ground lead) must be connected directly to the neutral electrode of the Hf-surgery equipment. Do not apply the other ECG electrodes too close to the operating area: **the distance must be at least 15 cm**. Measuring electrodes which could conduct the Hf-current away from the patient must not be attached to the patient during Hf-surgery.
- Keep unintentional current passageways (body trunk to extremities) dry by separating them with dry towels (Fig. 19.4). These towels should be changed from time to time during prolonged surgical procedures since they may become wet from the patient's sweat.

Equipment

- Hf-surgery equipment may be used only in rooms that have electrical installations that conform to national standards.

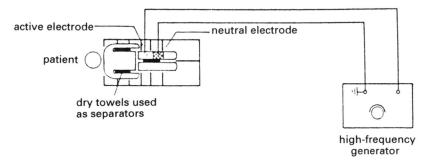

Fig. 19.4 Preventing unwanted current passages.

- Perform daily safety check as described previously.
- Place the foot switch so that it cannot be switched on by accident.
- Keep the electrode leads short and route them without forming sleeves (i.e. without crossing themselves or each other) and as far away as possible from other electrical cables. If other cables cross the Hf-electrode cables, high frequency may be transferred by induction into these cables, causing severe burns at their electrode connections to the patient.
- Use only intact cables approved by the manufacturer of the Hf-surgery equipment.
- **Always connect the neutral electrode first to the patient and then to the connector at the Hf-generator! The warning device of the Hf-generator indicates only that the neutral electrode cable is connected to the generator, not that it is connected to the patient. If it is connected first to the generator, the user might forget to connect it to the patient since the warning device will not indicate this.**

Hazards

For the user

- Burns caused by unintentional activation of the foot or hand switch (**watch out when changing electrodes**).
- Burns caused by moisture inside the electrode handle.
- Burns caused by a moisture bridge between unprotected hand and active electrode (**always wear insulating gloves when using Hf-surgery equipment**).
- Burns caused by touching metal parts with unprotected hands (during exchange of electrodes).
- Injuries caused by ignition of combustible gases, fumes or liquids near the application site of Hf-surgery.

For the patient

- Burns caused by unintentional activation of the Hf-surgery equipment.
- Burns caused by unsuitable operating table linings.
- Burns because of incorrect application of the neutral electrode.
- Burns within the region of the neutral electrode because of use of oxidized, bent, or dented metal plates, or by burns in neutral electrodes made of conductive rubber.

- Burns caused by contact with electrically conductive metal parts.
- Burns caused by ignition of combustible gases, fumes or liquids used near the application site of Hf-surgery.
- Burns caused by metallic parts fastened to or inside the body (metallic endoprostheses, etc.).
- Burns at the site of other electrodes attached to the body of the patient because of inductive Hf-currents (cable crossings with ECG cables, etc.).
- Burns at unintentional current bridges (body trunk to extremities).
- Electrolytic tissue damage caused by DC components added to the Hf-current.
- Interference with or failure of implanted cardiac pacemakers or the like.
- Interference with or failure of other important monitoring devices.
- Infections caused by unsuitably constructed electrode handle and switch.
- Damage to tissue outside the operating area caused by too high energy adjustment.
- Pressure necrosis caused by too tight fastening of the neutral electrode.

General remarks

Minor accidents caused by the use of Hf-surgery equipment are more common than generally believed. They are usually not recognized as accidents. For instance, burns caused by unintentional current bridges are not usually recognized as such because they do not resemble normal burns. Frequently, accidents caused by the user are blamed on the equipment (for instance necrosis caused by too tight fastening of the neutral electrodes).

References

von der Mosel, H.A. (1971a) Bioactive electrical signals, *Medical Electronics and Data* **2** (6), 68–71.
von der Mosel, H.A. (1971b) Electrical signals used for stimulation of muscular tissue, *Proc. Neuro-Electric Conference*, pp. 72–82, Charles C. Thomas, Springfield, Ill.
Quilligan, L. (1968) Induction of labour, *Hospital Practice* **11**, 44.

Further reading

Bayerisches Staatsministerium für Arbeit und Sozialordnung (1986) *Sichere Technik in der Medizin*, 2nd edn, pp. 32–36.

DIN VDE 0750 Teil 202 (1989) Besondere Fastlegungen für die Sicherheit von Hochfrequenz-Chirurgiegeräten.

DIN VDE 0753 Teil 1 (1983) Anwendungsregeln für Hochfrequenz-Chirurgiegeräte.

Hauser, K. (1990) Electrosurgery/laser surgery, *Medical Electronics* **21** (1), 162–164.

Hauser, K. (1990) Laser vs. electrosurgery: advantages and disadvantages, *Medical Electronics* **21** (1), 167.

Hauser, K. (1992) Electrosurgery/laser surgery, *Medical Electronics* **23** (1), 138–140.

Hauser, K. (1993) Electrosurgery, laser surgery, *Medical Electronics* **24** (1), 144–147.

Hauser, K. (1993) Endoscopic electrode safety, *Medical Electronics* **24** (2), 94–96.

Ministerium für Arbeit, Gesundheit und Soziales des Landes Nordrhein-Westfalen (1991) *Studie zur Verbesserung von Hochfrequenz-Chirurgiegeräten.*

Schlegel, H., Seipel, L. and Böhmighans, F. (1981) Funktionsstörungen von Demand-Schrittmachern bei urologischen Operationen mittels Elektrokauter, *Z. Kardiol.* **70**, 803.

Chapter 20
Infusion Pumps

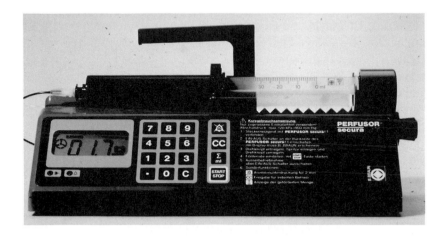

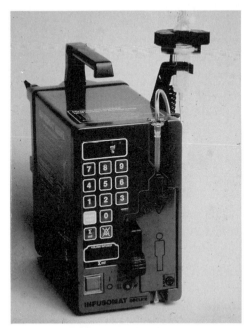

Syringe type of infusion pump (top) and infusion pump for larger quantities (base).

Principle of operation

Infusion pumps enable the pressure supported supply of liquids for parenteral nourishment; volume replacement; and the supply of electrolytes and medicine by means of sterile transfer systems through (preferably) venous admission to the patient.

Several safety provisions govern their function. In the event of faults, pumping will stop and an acoustic and optical alarm will be triggered.

Contrary to gravity infusion, infusion pumps are capable of overcoming flow resistance caused by pressure build-up within the system originating from high delivery rates, viscous solutions, tight catheters, cannulas and filters as well as that caused by movement of the patient. Hence, they warrant a higher degree of accuracy of delivery as well as an even flow throughout the duration of the infusion by maintaining the delivery rate as adjusted.

For the safe application of infusion pumps, the use of a hose system resistant to pressure is essential.

Infusion pumps are mainly applied when:

- a high volume accuracy is required, for instance for infusion of highly effective medicines (heparin, catecholamines, etc.),
- large volumes have to be infused within a short period of time,
- particularly small infusion quantities are required (for instance for keeping catheters open, etc.).
- exact quantities are to be supplied over a longer period of time.

Depending upon their mechanical principle of operation, three types of infusion pump can be differentiated.

- syringe-type infusion pumps,
- peristaltic hose pumps,
- piston or membrane pumps.

Syringe-type infusion pumps are used if small infusion quantities have to be delivered with a high degree of accuracy, as for instance with very potent medications, whereas the other types are used for larger infusion quantities.

Syringe-type infusion pumps

With this type of infusion pump, the infusion is performed by operating one or several syringes through a driving mechanism with a preselected speed. The delivery quantity is dependent upon the diameter of the syringe(s) and the speed of the syringe piston.

Peristaltic hose pumps

In peristaltic hose pumps a pump hose is squeezed by means of rollers or sliding bars, and the volume content within the hose is pushed towards the patient. According to the set delivery rate, the pump runs with more or less pumping cycles per unit of time. Depending upon construction, dosing is either drop or volume controlled.

In *drop-controlled pumps*, the number of drops per unit of time is counted by a drop sensor which controls the pump speed accordingly.

Volume-controlled pumps always deliver a constant volume per pump cycle to the patient. The delivery rate is determined exclusively by the rotational speed of the pump and the inner diameter of the transfer hose system used. The drop sensor is not necessary for this system; however, it is used for supervision, i.e. it triggers an alarm if, for example, the bottle containing the solution is empty and solution is no longer flowing.

Piston or membrane pumps

Among the volume-controlled infusion pumps there are also some types that have special pumping elements (volume chambers) such as piston or membrane pumps. The volume chambers are alternately filled and emptied through valves. Cycle number and filling volume of the chambers determine the delivery rate.

These pumps work with very high degree of precision, but the very elaborate disposable systems necessary for them are quite expensive.

Transfer systems

Drop-controlled infusion pumps can be operated using pressure-resistant standard hoses since the delivery tolerances of these hoses do not influence the accuracy of the drop regulation.

For volume-controlled infusion pumps, special pumping elements are necessary which have narrow internal diameter tolerances and are decisive for the accuracy of delivery of the pump.

The use of unsuitable pump hoses may cause uncontrolled flow of infusion solution to the patient. **Overdosages of up to 100% are possible despite properly functioning control systems.**

In syringe-type infusion pumps, the delivery rate depends upon the geometry of the syringe. **In order to avoid wrong dosage, only the syringe types recommended by the manufacturer must be used.**

On syringe pumps used with different types of syringe the drive speed is matched by inputting the code of the syringe geometry. However, the possible hazard of inputting the wrong code with the consequence of wrong dosage has to be considered.

Of major importance also is the safe fixation and correct insertion of the syringe into the pump. If the syringe pump is installed above the level of the patient, a hydrostatic pressure drop exists which causes suction within the transfer hose of the syringe. **In this case, if the syringe is not correctly inserted, or if the drive of the pump is not properly locked, the syringe may empty itself uncontrollably in a very short period of time.**

This suction may also cause entry of air into the patient through leaks in the syringe or at the connection of the transfer hose to the syringe. Both these situations might have serious consequences for the patient.

For safety reasons, only syringes and transfer hoses approved for the pump used must be used.

Relevant information can be found in the instruction manuals or on the packaging of the syringes and transfer hoses.

When using infusion pumps always make sure that not only the transfer system of the pump but also all system components such as filters, stopcocks and extension hoses withstand the pressure produced by the pump.

Control systems

Air control

Air infusion is a life-threatening hazard for the patient. In order to avoid its occurrence, infusion pumps have either a drop sensor that recognizes if the infusion bottle has run dry, or a sensor that checks the transfer hose, preferably at the pump exit, for air bubbles. Air bubbles that enter the hose system after it has left the pump can no longer be recognized by the pump.

In syringe-type infusion pumps, no air recognition systems are provided. The safety philosophy behind this type of infusion pump assumes that, as long as intact disposable systems are used and syringe and transfer hose are properly evacuated, no air can reach the patient.

Dosage control

In drop-controlled infusion pumps, the drop sensor will trigger an alarm even at very small deviations from the set drop rate.

In volume-controlled infusion pumps the drop sensor serves only for the control of empty infusion bottles, occlusion within the transfer system, or in massive free-flow situations. Control of dosage by means of the drop sensor is provided only rudimentarily in order to avoid false alarms.

Pressure control

In the event of occlusions within the system, kinked catheters or hoses, or erroneously closed stopcocks causing a rise in pressure within the system, infusion pumps will trigger an alarm as soon as a given pressure limit has been reached.

In hose pumps this is usually accomplished through the drop sensor which recognizes the non-appearance of the drop if the pump is no longer capable of delivering against the existing pressure.

In syringe-type pumps, the increased force necessary for the drive to work against the occlusion is used to recognize the over-pressure.

Since pressure changes below the alarm limits are interpreted by the pump as normal functions, disconnections or paravenous infusion will not be recognized.

Pumping capacity data of the pumps

Typical data on the pumping capacity of infusion pumps are:

- cut-off pressure,
- bolus,
- alarm delay time in the event of occlusion,
- discharge characteristics.

For syringe-type infusion pumps or pumps using silicone hoses or volume chambers, the *cut-off pressure* is about 1 bar or below.

Pumps using a PVC hose within the pumping area usually build up a pressure of about 3 bar and more. In the event of occlusion the pump will continue to deliver until the pressure alarm sounds, and hence will fill up the transfer system with the so-called *bolus pressure*.

As the occlusion opens, the bolus may reach the patient at full power. Depending upon the efficiency of the medication infused, the alarm delay time (the time from occlusion until triggering of the alarm) or even the bolus itself may be harmful to the patient.

It is important to prevent the bolus from reaching the patient.

The parameters pressure, bolus volume and alarm delay time are closely related to each other. The bolus volume increases with increasing pressure build-up and with increasing deformability of the transfer system. The *alarm delay time* depends upon the delivery rate. The alarm does not sound immediately but needs sufficient time to build up a bolus volume.

For therapy the conformity of the set rate to the effectively delivered rate is usually less important than the time stability of the delivery. The *discharge characteristics* of the different types of infusion pumps differ because of their different operational principles.

In syringe-type infusion pumps, a continuous volume flow is accomplished by even emptying of the syringe.

Piston-type pumps work continuously during the discharge phase of the volume chamber, interrupted by the standstill phase during the time the mini-syringe is refilled.

In peristaltic-type pumps, the volume flow changes periodically due to the pump head rotations. Observing the discharge characteristics within short time intervals, a continuously repeating over- and under-delivery will be observed while the average values of delivery correspond to the set delivery rate. If small delivery rates are used for highly potent medications that have short pharmacological half peak-value times, this discharge characteristic may be harmful to the patient. In this case, syringe-type infusion pumps are preferable.

To enable the user to make a judgement regarding the discharge characteristics of the pump to be used, the manufacturer should provide relevant information, usually in the form of advance cams (trumpet diagrams), in the instruction manual.

Equipment care

Infusion pumps must be cleaned and disinfected after every use. The information in the instruction manual must be followed carefully.

Under no circumstances should any liquid penetrate into the pump or its electrical connectors. Some pumps cannot be disinfected with alcoholic disinfectants since this might damage the material and inscriptions on the equipment. Always switch off the equipment and disconnect it from the electrical power line before cleaning and disinfecting it. Check visually for damage and external defects after every cleaning and disinfection.

In battery-operated infusion pumps, the batteries will discharge during longer storage periods. They must be recharged periodically, or they should be permanently connected to the electrical power line during storage.

Regular maintenance by a biomedical engineering technician or the manufacturer's service technician is necessary for safety reasons and to ensure that the equipment is permanently available.

Any dirt on the equipment housing caused by infusion solutions should be removed immediately to prevent it from drying on.

Daily safety check

Since infusion pumps are life-supporting equipment, they should be checked for safe function every day on which they are in use. The information in the instruction manual must be followed, and where such information is not provided, the manufacturer should be asked to provide it.

Most modern fusion pumps have an inbuilt self-testing facility. However, this self-test tests only the pump, not the connecting transfer systems. For this reason, all hoses must be checked for proper connections and to verify that they are capable of withstanding the pressure of the pump. For this purpose, the hose end towards the patient is closed with a clamp and the pump is started; no liquid should penetrate to the outside of the system, and the equipment must trigger an over-pressure alarm after a short while.

Before the pump is used again, check for the following:

- When is the next safety inspection due? If the time for this inspection is already overdue, do not use the pump before it is inspected.
- Is the equipment clean and correctly assembled?
- Has the equipment any recognizable damage? If so, it must not be used before repair.
- Make a visual inspection of power cord and connector for damage.
- Is the transfer hose system approved for this pump? Check also for damage (cracks, kinks, etc.).
- Is the battery fully charged?
- Is the delivery rate set properly?

Infusion pumps may be internally damaged after a fall even if no damage is visible. They should not be used before they are inspected by a bio-medical engineering technician.

Infusion pumps with any recognizable damage must not be used under any circumstances.

Application hints

Before an infusion pump is connected to a patient and switched on, always check once again in order to avoid possible harm to your patient:

- Safe position and safe attachment of the pump.
- Correct selection of the infusion solution.
- Is the infusion solution free of cloudiness and contamination?
- Is the infusion bottle free from damage?
- Is the correct transfer hose system or the correct syringe inserted?
- Is the transfer system free of air bubbles?
- Is the transfer hose system or the syringe inserted properly?
- During the use of the infusion pump on a patient, always check delivery rate and the contents level of the infusion bottle at regular intervals.

Remember: any fault you may miss in such an inspection might be very harmful to your patient!

Hazards

For the user

- Electrical shock caused by wet electrical connectors or damaged power cords.
- Injury from cannulas or sharp parts, with subsequent infection hazard.

For the patient

In addition to the potential hazards of infusion therapy generally (infections, incompatibility with medication, infusion of particles, etc.), the following risks exist for the patient from the use of infusion pumps:

- Air embolism.
- Blood loss caused by leakages within the system.
- Paravenous pressure infusion, tissue necroses.
- Hazards of electrical shock or caused by construction faults.
- Hazards caused by incorrect handling of the equipment, for instance massive overdoses if pump elements or syringes are wrongly inserted, etc.

Older infusion pumps that do not have pressure limiting devices should no longer be used because they have no alarm system and there is the hazard of rupture within the transfer system in the event of occlusion.

The use of several infusion pumps on the same patient requires special care. Bolus volume and alarm triggering time may vary considerably between the different pumps. If such a combination is absolutely necessary, only pumps of the same type and from the same manufacturer should be used together.

In combinations of peristaltic hose pumps that have different occlusion pressure characteristics, reflux is possible if the pump that has a stronger pressure overrides the mechanical occlusion pressure of the weaker pump.

Any combination of pump infusion and gravity infusion is extremely dangerous and should be avoided if possible.

In infusion therapy, never assume that everything will go well. The patient should be checked at regular intervals to ensure that all equipment is operating properly. This is particularly important in the case of combination infusions.

General remarks

Since infusion pumps are life-supporting and life-saving equipment, taking out a service contract with the manufacturer is strongly recommended.

Further reading

Abernathy, C.M. and Dickinson, T.C. (1979) Massive air embolism from intravenous infusion pump, *Amer. J. Surg.* **137**, 274.

Alexander, M.R., Kirking, D.M. and Baron, K.A. (1983) Utilization of electronic infusion devices in a university hospital, *Drug Intelligence and Clinical Nutrition* **3**, 630–633.

Anonymous (1990) Fluid delivery systems/pumps, *Medical Electronics* **21** (2), 178.

Anonymous (1992) Fluid delivery systems/pumps, *Medical Electronics* **23** (2), 149.

Auty, B. (1988) Equipment for intravenous infusion – some aspects of performance, *Agressologie* **29**, 824–828.

Auty, B. (1989) Controlled intravenous infusion – gravity feed or pumped systems? *Intensive Care World* **3** (9), 149–152.

Bayerisches Staatsministerium für Arbeit und Sozialordnung (1986) *Sichere Technik in der Medizin*, 2nd edn, pp. 46–48.

Clarkson, D. McG. (1992) Infusion pump performance testing, *Medical Electronics* **23** (2), 79–85.

Deterling, F. (1986) *Medizintechnik – Infusionstechnik*, Verlag TÜV, Rheinland.

DIN 58362 (1989) Transfusion, Infusion, Infusionsgeräte....

Fahey, P.J. (1990) Respirator care, ventilators, respirators, *Medical Electronics* **21** (1), 154–156.

Fahey, P.J. (1992) Respirator care, ventilators, respirators, *Medical Electronics* **23** (1), 125–127.

Ferenchak, P., Collins, J.J. and Morgan, A. (1971) Drop size and rate in parenteral infusion, *Surgery* **70**, 674.

Kelly, W.N. and Christensen, L.A. (1983) Selective patient criteria for the use of electronic infusion devices, *Amer. J. Intraven. Therapy Clin. Nutr.* **3**, 18–29.

Kindler, M. and Schuhmacher, W. (1988) Medizinische Gerätekunde: Infusionspumpen, *Die Schwester – Der Pfleger* **27** (7), 554–558.

Kreysch, W. (1984) *Praxis der Medizintechnik – Infusionsapparate*, Verlag TÜV Rheinland.

Motzkus, B. and Wolf, M. (1984) *Medizintechnik in Krankenhaus und Praxis: 1. Infusionsapparate*, Verlag de Gruyter, Berlin.

Tam, Y.C. (1989) Automated performance checking of infusion equipment, *Clin. Phys. Physiol. Meas.* **10**, 311–318.

Upton, J., Mullken, J.B. and Murray, J.E. (1979) Major intravenous extravasations injuries, *Amer. J. Surg.* **137**, 497–506.

Chapter 21
Electrotherapy Equipment

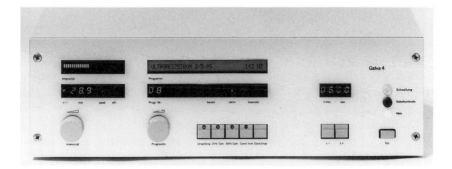

Example of electrotherapy machine.

Principle of operation

In the previous chapters about defibrillators and high-frequency surgical equipment we have discussed the influence of electrical current on biological tissues. All motor and neural processes within the human body are predominantly of electrical nature. Not only can these electrical processes be measured at the body surface (ECG, EEG, etc.); we can also influence them electrically from outside the body. There is thus a wide range of therapeutic possibilities for electrotherapy.

In electrotherapy, the required effect of electricity is accomplished by means of different forms of electrical current. These forms of current (DC, pulses, medium frequency diadynamic currents, etc.) have various effects on the biological mechanisms, i.e. each one of these current forms causes a specific effect within the organism.

Electrotherapy equipment can serve as a diagnostic tool (for instance for function tests of nerves and muscles) as well as for therapy (primarily for the treatment of diseases of the skeletal muscular system, in circulatory disturbances, conditions of pain of different origin, etc.). The effect is based on application of the electrical current directly to the patient which alters the resting potential of nerve and muscle cells (depolarization). This depolarization progresses through the nerve and muscle cells and causes, for instance, a muscle fibre to contract.

Since the effect of electrotherapy is based on electrical stimulation of tissues, it is also referred to as stimulation current therapy.

Diagnostic application of stimulation current (*I*/*t*-curve)

Diagnostic stimulation current is used mainly for examination of the nerve–muscle system. To test its excitability (RIC characteristics), *square waves* are used, and to examine its accommodation threshold as well as its degree of degeneration (DIC characteristic), *triangular pulses* are used.

Of great importance here is the recording of an *I*/*t* curve (*I* = stimulus intensity, *t* = stimulus duration). The evaluation of such a graph permits the reliable determination of suitable therapy as well as control of the progress of therapy.

The threshold values of muscular contraction in response to an electrical stimulation are particularly important as a means of determining the progress of electrotherapy.

Therapeutic application of stimulation currents

As already mentioned, different current forms have different effects on biological tissues.

DC (direct current, Fig. 21.1)

Constant (i.e. *not pulsating*) DC (galvanic current) is not a stimulation current in the true sense of the word. It does *not* produce stimulation of the cell. Its effect is based on alterations of the ionic environment caused by polarization within the tissues. It is only during switch-on and switch-off that a short stimulating effect exists which is caused by the exchange of K and Na ions through the cell membrane along the current pathway.

In physiotherapy, treatment using galvanization, i.e. with constant, not pulsating DC, is a commonly applied form of electrical current. Here, a DC (symbol =) of about 5 to 50 mA, depending upon the size of the electrodes, flows through the body tissues.

Galvanization has a circulation promoting, a pain reducing, a tonus regulating and an iontophoretic effect. The threshold of the receptors is increased.

The *circulation promoting* effect concerns skin and muscles. The hyperaemia improves the metabolic processes of the tissue.

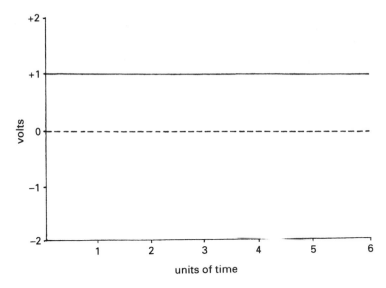

Fig. 21.1 Constant direct current.

The *pain reducing* effect is a consequence of the afore mentioned hyperaemia as well as of the damping of sensitive nerves in response to electrical effects.

The *tonus regulating* effect causes an improvement of the excitability of excitable structures, i.e. the capability of reacting to stimulation (stimulation current).

The *iontophoretic* effect permits percutaneous introduction of foreign ions, for instance medication, into the body.

Warning: Galvanization also has an electrolytic effect which may cause severe cauterization of the skin of the patient by OH ions where the electrode material comes into direct contact with the skin below the cathode. Cloth or sponges must therefore always be placed underneath the cathode.

Pulse currents (pulsating DC, Fig. 21.2)

Pulse currents are true stimulating currents. Periodical on-and-off switching causes repeated exchange of K and Na ions through the cell membrane. That is, the resting potential of nerve or muscle cells is constantly depolarized and repolarized. The cells react to these electrical stimuli, for example by contraction (at switching on of the current) and relaxation (at switching off of the current). The actual effect of such

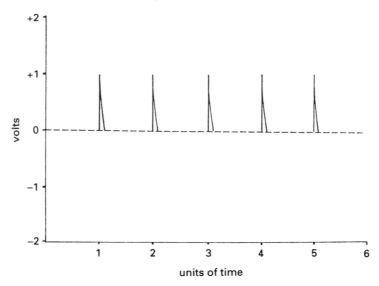

Fig. 21.2 Pulsating direct current.

pulses on the cells depends upon the speed of the pulse sequence (frequency):

- A single pulse causes a short muscle contraction (Tic) followed by immediate relaxation. Even at frequencies of 1–5 Hertz (1–5 pulses/second), a (still) full relaxation follows every (still) full contraction of the muscle.
- At pulse frequencies from 5 to about 20 Hertz (5– 20 pulses/second), the time between the single pulses is too short to accomplish full relaxation. An incomplete tetany, also called *shake frequency*, is the result.
- At pulse frequencies of more than 30 Hertz (more than 30 pulses/second), the muscle remains in tetany since the pulses follow each other faster than a full relaxation can be accomplished. The single contractions add up to a complete contraction of the muscle fibre.

Among pulse currents, different pulse shapes can be differentiated, for example square pulses, triangular pulses, exponential pulses (also called saw-tooth pulses), half-wave pulses, etc.

The essential characteristic of pulse currents is that they always go only from zero-volt to plus-volt values or, depending on their polarity, from zero-volt to minus-volt values and back. They are DC not AC (alternating current) pulses.

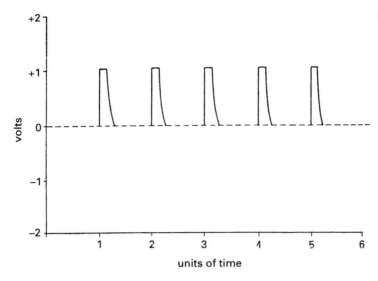

Fig. 21.3 Square pulses.

In physiotherapy, it is primarily the following pulse shapes that are applied.

Square pulses (Fig. 21.3)

Square pulses are used, for example, as *ultrastimulation current* (Traebert ultrastimulation) for stimulation current massage, mainly in cases of accidental injuries in the region of the spine, and where there are pathological changes of the bones, etc. For more details see Steuernagel (1984).

Half-wave pulses (Fig. 21.4)

According to Bernard, half-wave pulses are applied as *diadynamic currents* for the treatment of pain conditions, the acceleration of oedema resorption, detonization of hypertonic and contracted muscles, and reduction of the sympaticotonus, and to damp sympaticus caused pain conditions. For more details see Gillman (1982) and Steuernagel (1984).

Alternating current (AC, Fig. 21.5)

AC of medium frequency (1 to 100 kilohertz) has been used in

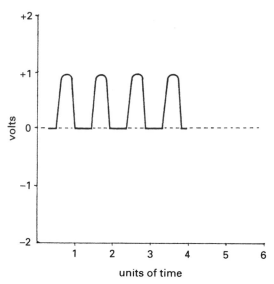

Fig. 21.4 Half-wave pulses.

physiotherapy since 1957. Compared with similar low frequency pulses, it has several advantages:

- Patients perceive it as more pleasant.
- It permits blockage of stimulus propagation in nerves.
- It enables specific testing of Head and Mackenzie zones. For more details see Boegelein (1991) and Steuernagel (1984).

Electrotherapy is frequently combined with suction massage or with ultrasound therapy.

Suction massage

The effect is increased owing to the summation of stimuli. At the same time, the patient perceives this combination as more pleasant.

Ultrasound therapy

For information on the combination of electrotherapy with ultrasound therapy (simultaneous method) see Chapter 23.

It is not the role of this book to discuss the electronic principles of production of the different current forms and frequencies.

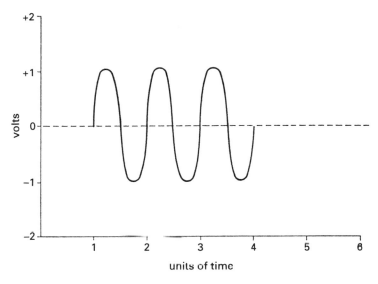

Fig. 21.5   Alternating current.

Equipment care

Care of electrotherapy equipment is simple and is limited to the following which, however, must be done after *every* use of the equipment:

- Always keep metallic electrodes clean and shiny. Oxidation at the patient contact areas (seen as greyish staining) increases resistance to electrical current and hence may reduce the effectively delivered amount of current. The surfaces must be cleaned with a good metal polish until they are shiny.
- After iontophoresis, residues of the medication used must be carefully removed from the electrodes and the sponges.
- Rubber bells from suction massage electrodes should be treated, from time to time, with glycerine or Vaseline in order to prevent them from getting brittle.
- Alligator clips for connection of disposable electrodes should be regularly cleaned, particularly on the inner side. Electrode gel residues can easily be removed by means of a needle.
- Check electrode cables every week for cracks or breaks in the insulation. If these are present, renew the cables immediately.
- Check connectors for shaky contacts which could cause a sudden high current shock to the patient.
- Check from time to time that all control lamps and meters are

working properly. If not, have them repaired immediately since otherwise you cannot ensure the effective delivery of the parameters you have set.

- Check for any additional care instructions from the manufacturer.

Daily safety check

Unfortunately, very few manufacturers have so far described how such a test is to be done. The user is strongly recommended to ask the manufacturers for details.

Always bear in mind that, in the event of an accident, the user/owner will be held responsible.

Application hints

- Let the equipment have some warm-up time before using it on a patient.
- First, set all controls to zero.
- Select the required programme.
- Position your patient comfortably.
- Clean the skin well at the application sites.
- Moisten electrode sponges using tap water (no saline solution). If you use suction electrodes make sure that the sponges are not too wet so that no water can penetrate into the suction massage equipment.
- Do not place electrodes over projecting bones with little muscular cover or above skin defects or metallic implants, close to eczematous areas, or over oedematous soft tissue swellings.
- Electrodes must be placed firmly on the skin. However, do not fasten rubber straps too tightly.
- In galvanization, use disposable electrodes only with special care (danger of hydrolysis).
- Pay special attention in galvanization that no direct skin contact exists with electrode material or metallic electrode connectors, even if the patient should move.
- Turn current strength up *slowly*. The current strength should not cause unpleasant sensations for the patient.
- Before changing the programme or the polarity, turn all controls back to zero.
- At the end of treatment, first reset all controls back to zero, then disconnect the electrodes from the patient, and only then switch off the equipment.

- After *every* use, take the electrode sponges from the electrodes and disinfect them. Wipe metallic electrodes dry in order to avoid oxidation.
- In iontophoresis, make sure that the medication is applied **at the correct polarity**.
- After iontophoresis, always remove all residual medication from electrodes and sponges.
- Check polarity carefully in galvanization.
- Never use electrotherapy equipment close to Hf-surgery equipment, diathermy and microwave equipment, or radio transmitters. These must be at least 6 metres away.
- Use only electrodes and electrode cables approved by the manufacturer.
- Never use electrotherapy equipment near inflammable gases, etc.
- In interference treatment using two pairs of electrodes, do not intertwine the electrode cables into 'plaits'. Induction and undesired and uncontrollable currents may be produced within the cables.
- In order to avoid possible secondary accidents, there should be no sharp-cornered furniture near the patient.

Hazards

For the user

- Weak electric shocks caused by unintentional contact with the electrodes, damaged insulation of electrode cables, and possible transfer of electricity from the patient to nearby metallic furniture or equipment, particularly if the user has moist hands.
- Secondary accidents following electrical shocks (caused by fright, subsequent fast withdrawal and knocking against a sharp corner).

For the patient

Injuries can be caused by disregarding contra indications.

Absolute contra indications

- Inflammations.
- Diseases accompanied by fever (reduced skin resistance caused by sweating).
- Acute purulent processes.
- Tumour-suspicious processes.
- Tuberculosis.

- Advanced arteriosclerosis.
- Haemorrhages and the tendency to haemorrhage.
- Parkinson's disease.
- Progressive muscular dystrophy.
- Amyotrophic lateral sclerosis.
- Essential spastic spinal paralysis.
- Implanted cardiac pacemakers.

Localized contra indications

- Application of DC or galvanic pulse currents near metallic implants.
- Within the abdominal and lumbar region during pregnancy.
- Abdominally during menstruation.
- Thromboses.
- Thrombophlebitis.
- In eczemamatous areas (except iontophoresis).

Relative contra indications

- In poliomyelitis **no electrotherapy during the acute state**. Electrotherapy may be started (against muscular atrophy) during the first week of reconvalescence (after about 3 to 6 months).
- No stimulation current in case of myotonic or myasthenic reactions.
- In multiple sclerosis during acute attacks.
- In case of apoplexies of other vascular origins if, following electrotherapy, the blood pressure rises more than 20 mmHg. Measurement is necessary before and after electrotherapy.
- Special attention (limitation of current intensity) in case of hypoaesthesias and anaesthesias.
- Consider the possibility of allergies in iontophoresis!
- Transthoracic heart stimulation current only with low intensity, motoric below threshold.
- If too high a current intensity is used in cranial galvanization, the occurrence of the Ménière symptom complex is possible.

References

Boegelein, K. (1991) *Mittelfrequenz-Fibel,* Verlag Zimmer Elektromedizin, Neu-Ulm.

Gillmann, H. (1982) *Physikalische Therapie – Grundlagen und Wirkungsweisen,* G. Thieme Verlag, Stuttgart.

Steuernagel, O. (1984) *Skripten zur Elektrotherapie,* 9th ed, Vols I and II Selbstverlag des Verfassers, Boppard a. Rhein.

Further reading

Anonymous (1990) Stimulators (muscle/nerve/TENS), *Medical Electronics* **21** (4), 159–161.

Cady, R.K. and Shealy, C.N. (1990) Electrotherapy in medicine, *Medical Electronics* **21** (1), 122–128.

Closson, W.J. (1985) Transcutaneous electrical nerve stimulation and ACTH production, *Amer. J. Electromedicine* **1** (3), 7.

Comeau, M. and Brummet, R. (1978) Anesthesia of the human tympanic membrane by iontophoresis of a local anesthetic, *Laryngoscope* **88**, 277.

DIN VDE 0750 Teil 219 (1989) Medizinische elektrische Geräte; besondere Festlegung für die Sicherheit von Reizstromgeräten für Nerven und Muskeln.

Dirschauer, A. *et al.* (1980) *Physikalische Therapie in Klinik and Praxis*, Kohlhammer Verlag, Stuttgart.

Drago, G.P. and Ridella, S. (1982) Evaluation of electrical fields inside a biological structure, *Brit. J. Cancer* **45** Suppl. V, 215–219.

Edel, M. (1977) *Fibel der Elektrodiagnostik und Elektrotherapie*, 4th edn, Steinkopf Verlag, Dresden.

Friedenberg, Z.B., Harlow, M.C., and Brighton, C.T. (1974) Healing of non-union of the medial malleolus by means of direct current: a case report, *J. Trauma* **11**, 883–884.

Jantsch, H. (1980) Mittelfrequente Reizströme, *Zeitschr. Phys. Med.* **2**, 137–140.

von der Mosel, H.A. (1971) Electrical signals used for stimulation of muscular tissues, in *Neuroelectric Research*, Charles C. Thomas, Springfield, Ill, 72–82.

Shatin, D. Surface electrical stimulation for the treatment of idiopathic scoliosis, *New Frontiers in TENS*, Hymes, A.C. (Ed.), Chapter 17.

Shealy, C.N. (1967) Electrical inhibition of pain by stimulation of the dorsal column: preliminary clinical reports, *Anesth. Analg. (Cleveland)* **45**, 489.

Shealy, C.N. (1974) Transcutaneous electrical stimulation for control of pain, *Clin. Neurosurg.* **21**, 269–277.

Shealy, C.N. (1975) The viability of external electrical stimulation as a therapeutic modality, *Medical Instrumentation* **9**, 5.

Sisler, H.A. (1978) Iontophoresis local anesthesia for conjunctival surgery, *Ann. Ophthalm.* **10**, 597.

Svarcova, J., Trnavsky, K. and Zvarova, J. (1988) The influence of ultrasound, galvanic currents, and shortwave diathermy on pain intensity in patients with osteoarthrosis, *Scand. J. Rheumatol.* **67**, 83–85.

Chapter 22
Premature Baby Incubators

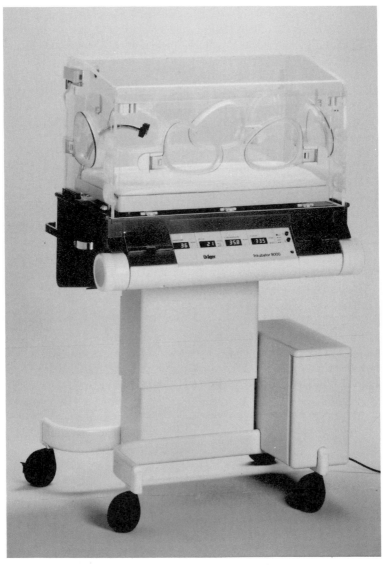

Typical baby incubator.

Principle of operation

The premature baby incubator is a very important piece of intensive care equipment for use in newborn baby units. It provides a protective environment for premature babies and hence improves their chances of survival. This protective environment is provided in order to avoid, as much as possible, stressing their still unstable thermoregulation system, and to keep their energy requirements for maintaining their body temperature as low as possible. This also means a lower oxygen requirement.

Compared with normal babies born at the correct time, the body surface of premature babies is considerably larger in relation to their body weight. As a result their heat production per cm^2 body surface is smaller although the heat losses through the body surface are very high, particularly for these patients. The incubator is provided to help to compensate for this special stress. However, this is possible only if all heat transport mechanisms are combined in such a way as to produce this protective environment.

The protective environment includes the correct temperature, the correct concentration of oxygen within the room air for the respiration of the baby, and the maintenance of the correct air humidity. Naturally, the protective environment must also be free of infectious bacteria.

Although the principle of operation of this kind of equipment is actually easy to understand, a relatively large number of accidents occur when using it because some of the technical functions of the equipment are not properly understood.

Temperature

The (adjustable) temperature of the interior of an incubator should remain as stable as possible, including during working conditions, i.e. if the working windows of the hood are open. Warmth is the actual purpose of care of premature babies within an incubator. Depending on the manufacturer, the measures range from heat curtains between double walls, through radiation heat, to convection heating. All these measures have one thing in common: the temperature around the patient is regulated by thermostats. These are electronic components which switch the heater off as soon as the set temperature is reached, and switch the heater on again as soon as the temperature goes below the set level. **However, these thermostats affect only the heaters built into the incubator!**

There have been repeated reports of overheating of the interior of the incubator and hence also of the patient. In such cases death is often the result. These incidents were caused by well meaning nurses who inserted an additional heating blanket or the like into the incubator. Since such additional heaters are not switched on or off by the incubator's thermostat, overheating of the interior of the incubator results even though the thermostats correctly turn off the incubator's built-in heater. **Additional heat sources and other accessories which are not specifically provided for the particular type of incubator must never be used inside the incubator!**

Other heat sources such as sunshine through a nearby window; room heaters near the incubator, phototherapy equipment, etc. can influence the temperature inside the incubator uncontrollably. This must therefore be borne in mind when deciding where to place the incubator within the ward. **Phototherapy lamps and the hood of the incubator must not be covered with blankets, tinfoil or the like in order to enhance the effects of phototherapy. This would cause heat localization since the absolutely necessary cooling effect of the surrounding air would be lost.**

Despite all the temperature controls built into the incubator it is absolutely essential that the nurse on duty inspects the incubator for correct temperature at regular intervals!

Oxygen

Enrichment of oxygen in the respiration air inside the incubator must be done **strictly according to the physician's prescription only!** It must be controlled only according to the oxygen partial pressure measured in the arterial blood of the patient. Only in this way is it possible to prevent hyperoxaemia, which would endanger the eyes (retrolental fibroplasia) and hypoxaemia, which would damage the patient's brain.

If the air is enriched with oxygen, note the possible fire hazard. No source of ignition such as an open fire, matches, lit cigarettes or the like must be used in rooms where incubators are in use. In an atmosphere enriched with oxygen, textiles, oils and plastics are easily inflammable and burn with high intensity.

Humidity of air

The frequently underestimated heat losses caused by evaporation call for particular attention. Of special concern are the water losses of very small premature babies; considerable quantities of water can diffuse through their skin (see Fig. 22.1). Since the body loses 560 kilocalories of heat energy with every gramme of diffused water, this loss of heat is a very decisive factor if premature babies of low gestation age are to be

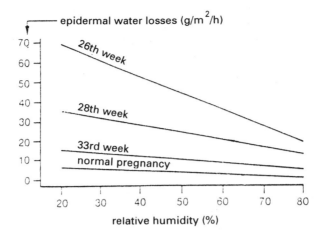

Fig. 22.1 Relationship of water loss and atmospheric humidity.

kept warm during their first days of life. For this reason, transepidermal water losses should be reduced as much as possible. This is the reason why, in incubators, the air humidifying system is always a central part of the protective environment.

The capability of air to absorb water vapour is very high, particularly at high temperatures. Room air at a temperature of 25°C, even if it has a relative humidity of 50%, has only a relative humidity of 25% left if warmed up to 37°C. If oxygen is added, the conditions are even more unfavourable: here, the relative humidity will be only 10% in the event of the same increase of heat as above (see Fig. 22.2).

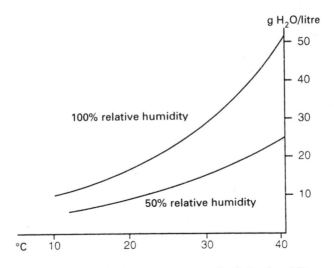

Fig. 22.2 Relationship of room temperature and relative humidity.

For reasons of hygiene, waterbath-type air humidification systems are seldom used. Hence the air inside the incubator is frequently too dry, causing the transepidermal water losses to be too high as well. If distilled and sterilized water is used in the right quantities, and if the water tank is properly sterilized after cleaning, concern on the grounds of hygiene is no longer justified.

The rule of thumb in order to achieve the correct level of air humidification is: do not apply any extreme combinations of temperature/humidity, but combine high air humidity with higher air temperatures. On the other hand, for larger patients, a lower incubator temperature should be combined with a lower humidity. In addition, the humidity should be adjusted in such a way that condensation on the walls of the incubator hood (which is undesirable for optical as well as for hygiene reasons) is just avoided.

To summarize, it is the task of the incubator to provide the correct, protective environment for babies. It is vital that the user understand all the components necessary; the user must also be fully aware of the correct combination of the different components.

Furthermore it is absolutely essential that the user check regularly the components of the incubator which produce the correct protective environment. **Never forget that even the best technology may fail! As well as technical failure it is important to bear in mind the possibility of human failure.**

Equipment care

As already mentioned, the premature baby incubator is life-saving equipment. Its reliable functioning is of greatest importance for the survival of premature babies. This means that the equipment must be regularly inspected and maintained. **Taking out a service contract with the manufacturer is highly recommended.**

Regular care by nursing staff is limited to cleaning, sterilization and visual inspection for damage, breaks, ruptures, etc., of the connecting hoses, the incubator hood and the electrical connecting cable, as well as ensuring correct assembly after cleaning and sterilization. Before every application check that the assembly condition corresponds to the case specific therapeutic requirements (respirator, body temperature sensor, etc.).

After *every* change of patient and *at least once weekly* the incubator must be cleaned and disinfected thoroughly. Disinfection must be performed according to the manufacturer's recommendations.

After disinfection and reassembly, the incubator must be

switched on and must run for several hours to evaporate residual disinfectant completely in order to avoid its inhalation by the patient.

If a new fresh filter is inserted, always note the date of insertion. Such filters must be renewed at least every 2 months. Make sure when inserting the filter that it covers the entire fresh air inlet and is inserted correctly (the arrow on the edge of the filter must point towards the interior of the incubator).

Daily safety check

This test should be performed according to the manufacturer's instructions. Some of the newer incubators have an in-built self-testing function. If there is no mention of this test in the instruction manual and the incubator does not have self-testing functions, the test must be performed as follows:

- Visual inspection to check that the incubator is assembled correctly (see instruction manual!).
- Check the date of insertion and the correct insertion of the fresh air filter.
- Check contents level of the air humidifier. Always have sufficient sterile distilled water ready.
- Are all cables and hoses correctly installed and routed?
- Is the incubator properly connected to the power supply?
- Are all uncontrollable heat sources (sunlight, room heater, etc.) far enough away from the incubator?
- Is the oxygen supply correctly connected? If oxygen gas bottles are used, check how full they are and make sure you have spares available.
- Close oxygen valve and check oxygen fault alarm. Reopen oxygen valve.
- Check that the oxygen meter is functioning properly.
- Remove power line connector from the electrical wall outlet. Does the power failure alarm work properly? Reconnect power line connector to the wall outlet.
- Test over-temperature and under-temperature alarms and ventilator failure alarm.
- Disconnect skin temperature sensor and check that the sensor fault alarm is working properly. Reconnect it.
- Test air humidity control and indicator.
- Are all parameters correctly set according to the physician's prescription for the next patient?

These checks must be repeated *daily* as far as this is possible without endangering the patient (see instruction manual or ask the manufacturer).

Application hints

- Before every application of the incubator, always perform the safety check as described above.
- Before any use of the incubator for a new patient, always prewarm it for at least 35 minutes.
- Check several times a day that the incubator is not exposed to sunlight in order to avoid uncontrolled heating of the interior.
- Before phototherapy is applied, always reduce the incubator's interior temperature by about 2°C.
- The skin temperature of the patient is a good criterion for the correct temperature adjustment of the incubator.

  Warning: do not adjust the temperature of the interior of the incubator according to the patient's skin temperature in cases of trauma or similar conditions.

- As in all intensive care units, patient and equipment (incubator) require constant supervision. Never rely on the inbuilt alarm systems alone. Technology can fail occasionally.
- Make it a habit to check the correct setting of temperature, oxygen supply and air humidity every time you have done some work in or at the incubator.
- Note the higher demand for air humidity if oxygen is used (see Fig. 22.2).
- Never use the alarm suppression to complete other work without disturbance! **If an alarm sounds, always react at once!**
- Inspect regularly the correct position of the skin temperature sensor. It may get displaced or even detached if the patient moves.
- Check very carefully the physician's prescribed oxygen dosage in order to avoid permanent harm to the patient. Check regularly the actual oxygen concentration administered to the patient.
- The rectal temperature of the patient must be controlled permanently **in addition to the skin temperature**, particularly during the first hours of incubator care.
- If the front plate of the incubator is open, the patient must be constantly supervised in order to prevent him or her from falling out!

- Bear in mind that the room temperature has a considerable influence on the temperature inside the incubator. This applies particularly if phototherapy is applied!
- Admission of liquids, for example by parenteral infusion, must be increased during phototherapy, because this leads to increased water demand as the child will sweat more.
- For CPAP patients the respiration gas temperature must be permanently controlled since the respiration gas hoses may get warmed up by the warmed circulating incubator air.
- The rated value of the air temperature adjustment should be increased over 37°C only on the express orders of the physician. If this is done, the patient's temperature must be monitored particularly carefully.
- After every change of patient, or at least once a week, the incubator must be cleaned and sterilized.
- Switch on the incubator for several hours after every sterilization so that residual disinfectant can evaporate fully. It is poisonous to the patient!
- Always bear in mind that premature babies are very sensitive patients and hence need very careful supervision. It is for this reason that the application hints have been treated in such detail.

Hazards

For the patient

- Overheating of the interior of the incubator may cause death of the patient.
- Too high heat loss as a result of transepidermal water loss caused by too low air humidity.
- Irreparable eye damage (retrolental fibroplasia) caused by hyperoxaemia due to too high oxygen concentration in the respiration air inside the incubator.
- Irreparable brain damage caused by hypoxaemia due to too low oxygen concentration in the respiration air inside the incubator.
- Increased fire hazard during oxygen application.
- Poisoning of the patient caused by disinfectant residues present within the incubator.
- Danger of infection of the patient due to insufficient sterilization of the incubator.

General remarks

As already noted, an unacceptably high number of accidents during the use of baby incubators have been reported internationally. These accidents were almost exclusively caused by the users. Reference is made to the examples of accidents given in Chapter 3.

Further reading

Ad-Hoc-Kommission des Bundesgesundheitsamtes (1985) Zweite Emfehlung der Ad-Hoc-Kommission des Bundesgesundheitsamtes: Formaldehyd in Inkubatoren, *Bundesgesundheitsblatt* **28** (5).

Alm, A. and Bill, A. (1972) The oxygen supply to the retina, *Acta physiol. Scand.* **84**, 261, 306.

Bauer, C.R. and Windmayer, S. (1981) A relationship between p_aO_2 and retrolental fibroplasia, *Pediatr. Res.* **15**, 649.

Baumgart, S. and Engle, W.D. (1981) Effect of heat shielding on corrective and evaporative heat losses and on radiant heat transfer in the premature infant, *J. Pediatr.* **99** (6), 940.

Bell, E.F. *et al.* (1980) The effects of thermal environment on heat balance and insensible water loss in low birth-weight infants, *J. Pediatr.* **96**, 452–459.

DIN VDE 0750 Teil 212 (1987) *Medizinische elektrische Geräte Säuglingsinkubatoren – Besondere Festlegungen für die Sicherheit*, Beuth Verlag, Berlin.

DIN VDE 0750 Teil 217 (1987) *Medizinische elektrische Geräte – Transportinkubatoren – Besondere Festlegungen für die Sicherheit*, Beuth Verlag, Berlin.

Frankenberger, H. and Güthe, A. (1991) *Inkubatoren*, Verlag TÜV Rheinland, Cologne.

Hammerlund, K. and Sendin, G. (1979) Transepidermal water loss in newborn infants, III: relation to gestational age, *Acta Paediatr. Scand.* **68**, 795–801.

Hey, E. (1969) The relation between environmental temperature and oxygen consumption in the newborn baby, *J. Physiol.* **200**, 589.

Hey, E. and Katz, G. (1970) The optimum thermal environment for naked babies, *Arch. Dis. Childh.* **45**, 328.

Korones, S.B. (1986) *High Risk Newborn Infants – The Basis for Intensive Nursing Care*, 4th edn, C.V. Mosby Company, St Louis.

LeBlanc, M.H. (1987) The physics of thermal exchange between infants and their environment, *Med. Instrumentation* **21** (1), 11–15.

McDonald, A.D. (1964) Oxygen treatment of premature babies and cerebral palsy, *Developm. Med. Child Neurol.* **6**, 313.

Obladen, M. (1987) Thermoregulation und Thermoregulationsstörungen bei Neugeborenen, in *Beitr. Intensiv-Notfall Med.*, Vol. 6, pp. 82–99, Karger Verlag, Basel.

Okken, A. *et al.* (1984) Insensible water loss and metabolic rate in low birth-weight newborn infants, *Pediatr. Res.* **13**, 1072–1075.

Terry, T.L. (1942) Extreme prematurity and fibroplastic overgrowth of persistent vascular sheath behind each crystalline lens, preliminary report, *Amer. J. Ophthalm.* **25**, 203.

Chapter 23
Ultrasonic Therapy Equipment

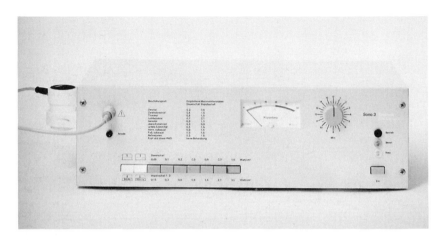

Example of ultrasound therapy equipment.

Principle of operation

The frequency range of sound which is audible to the human ear is between 60 Hertz and 20 kilohertz (= 20 000 Hertz). Sound at a frequency above 20 kilohertz cannot be recognized by the human ear and is called ultrasound.

If an AC current flows through a piezoelectric material such as lead zirconate, the material changes in size according to the rhythm of the frequency current applied. This makes it a 'mechanical oscillator'. Ultrasound therapy is the application of mechanical oscillation (sound) within the ultrasonic range of frequency for therapeutic purposes. It is applied primarily for the treatment of painful changes within the skeleton as well as to the muscle–tendon system.

Ultrasonic waves can only propagate in the presence of mass particles within a medium. They are not conducted through air or in a vacuum. For this reason a coupling medium has to be applied between the source of sound (the sound head) and the tissue to be treated with ultrasonic energy. If by chance the sound head is tilted during treatment, i.e. if it is

198

not held level with the surface of the skin, ultrasound will be transmitted to the tissue only from the part of the sound head that is in direct contact with the coupling medium and the tissue. An incorrect dosage of applied ultrasonic energy will be the result.

With increasing depth, ultrasonic energy is absorbed by the tissues. This absorption differs in intensity depending upon the conditions of the tissues. Bone tissue absorbs ultrasonic energy ten times better than muscular tissue, and this in turn absorbs it 2.5 times better than fatty tissues. Tendons, ligaments and joint capsules do absorb more ultrasonic energy than do the tissues of epidermis, the panniculum and muscular tissues.

The mechanical energy of ultrasound is transformed primarily into heat depending on the absorption capability of the tissue and on other factors. Therapeutically usable heat will be generated by an applied energy level of about 0.05 watts per cm^2 (= 50 mW/cm^2).

The peculiarity of the heat distribution spectrum of ultrasonic energy is the selective heating of interphases, particularly those where media of different resistance against sound waves (impedance) meet. This applies to the interphase between bones and muscles.

If the ultrasonic energy dose is too high, it may cause harmful mechanical effects originating from cavitation (formation of cavities). If, however, the recommended energy dose is selected; if the presently customary technique involving the use of a moving – not stationary – sound head is applied (dynamic acoustic irradiation); if contra-indications are properly regarded; and if the equipment is in the correct condition, such impairments can safely be avoided.

Equipment care

Ultrasonic therapy equipment needs little care by the user. The following, however, should be carried out regularly.

- Test proper function of the equipment daily before its first use (see next section).
- After *every* patient, clean the sound head carefully of all residues of the coupling medium, using alcohol or methylated spirit.
- Clean the equipment housing whenever necessary using a damp (*not wet*) cloth.
- Check all cables and connectors for damage from time to time.
- **Even if you regard yourself as a good technician, never try to 'repair' any part of this equipment yourself!**

The equipment should be maintained and recalibrated by the manufacturer or his authorized service organization at least every second
year.

Daily safety check

Every day before first use check the equipment for proper function. This
should be done as follows:

- Hold the sound head in such a way that its radiating surface points
  upwards.
- Using an eye dropper (pipette), apply slowly just sufficient water on
  its surface that about three-quarters of it is covered.
- Switch on the equipment and select, in sequence, the following
  energy levels:

  0.1 W/cm^2:   You should see a slight bubbling of the water such as is
  seen in sparkling mineral water.

  0.5 W/cm^2:   The water should now look as if boiling although it is
  cold.

  1.0 W/cm^2:   Water particles should shoot explosively from the
  radiating surface.

If, during this test, the water should behave differently, the power
selector may be out of calibration. **In this case, it is strongly recommended that the equipment is not used until the manufacturer's
service technician has checked it.**

Note: The safety check as described above is *not* a calibration. It only
serves the purpose of checking whether or not the equipment appears to
be functioning properly.

Application hints

- Place the patient comfortably and in a relaxed position for treatment.
- Cold extremities should be warmed up before treatment in order to
  avoid the stimulative effects of the coldness.
- For the same reason, the coupling medium should be warmed up to
  body temperature before it is applied to the patient.
- For underwater treatment the water should be free of air bubbles.
  Also, air bubbles covering hairy parts of the patient's body should be
  carefully removed before treatment.
- Make sure to exclude the possibility of contraindications before the
  patient is treated. If in doubt call the physician.

- Never exceed the ultrasonic energy level as prescribed by the physician.
- Avoid tilting the sound head during treatment. It must always be flat on the body surface.
- During treatment pay attention to possible signs of overdose.
- At the end of therapy the patient should rest for at least 30 minutes before leaving. Driving a motor vehicle immediately after treatment might be dangerous!

Hazards

Ultrasonic therapy is by no means as harmless as generally believed. Pay attention particularly to contraindications, but a number of other facts also have to be borne in mind.

For the user

- In case of 'indirect coupling' of the sound head (underwater treatment), the hand of the therapist guiding the sound head might be exposed unintentionally to ultrasonic radiation as a result of reflective processes (for instance from the tub wall, etc.). To avoid this:

  ○ Use a tub of sufficient size.
  ○ Wear two pairs of rubber gloves.
  ○ Fasten the sound head to a carrying arm and move it with this under water instead of using your hands directly.

- In water therapy, a sound head with damage to its watertight housing may leak electrical current into the water (electrical shock hazard!).

For the patient

Contraindications

- Acute inflammatory processes, fever, acute diseases.
- Tuberculosis, bronchiectases.
- Vascular diseases of the extremities such as thrombophlebitis, thrombosis, varicosis, haemorrhagic diathesis.
- Pre- and postoperative malign and benign tumours.
- Circulatory insufficiency, coronary diseases, irregularities of the cardiac rhythm.
- Neuralgias of unknown genesis.

- Abnormalities of blood coagulation.
- Acute polyarthritis.
- Progressed peripheral arterial circulatory disturbances (stage III and IV according to Fontaine).
- Patients up to 8 months after completion of ionization therapy.
- Diseases for which heat is a contraindication. In such cases, careful treatment at an energy level not exceeding 0.05 W/cm^2 is permissible.
- Be extremely careful with patients who have an implanted cardiac pacemaker! Ultrasonic energy applied directly over the location of the pacemaker or its connecting cable to the heart may cause breakage of the soldering joints of the pacemaker or breakage of the cable.

Ultrasonic therapy must not *be applied to:*

- Eyes.
- Testicles, ovaries, uterus during pregnancy.
- Epiphyseal lines.
- Laminectomy scars.
- Large organs such as liver, spleen, lung.
- Higher segments than C3 paravertebrally.

Ultrasonic therapy must be applied with care *to:*

- Bone projections covered by only little soft tissues.
- Patients suffering from advanced vegetative dystony.
- Patients suffering from advanced arteriosclerosis.
- Patients in generally poor condition.
- Children generally.
- Do not treat anaesthetized areas of patients who have impaired sensitivity since symptoms of overdose (pain) cannot be recognized.

Further possible sources of hazard

- Electrical shock hazard in underwater treatment (indirect coupling) if sound head is no longer watertight.
- Wrong ointments used as coupling medium may produce too much heating and even burns.
- Too high an ultrasonic energy level can cause cavitation (irreversible tissue damage, tissue rupture, acidosis).
- Overheating of sound head if activated without tissue contact for any extended period of time.
- After the first few therapy sessions, central nervous problems

(headache, dizziness, tiredness, circulatory problems, etc.) may occur. Patients should not therefore drive a motor vehicle immediately after treatment.

General remarks

Keep ultrasonic therapy equipment at least 5 metres away from diathermy, microwave and high-frequency surgical equipment and from radio transmitters.

Further reading

Anonymous (1990) Ultrasound, *Medical Electronics* **21** (3), 142–143.

Edel, H. and Boegelein, K. (1989) *Ultrasound Primer*, Zimmer Elektromedizin Corp., Irvine, CA.

Knoch, H.G. and Knauth, K. (1972) *Therapie mit Ultraschall*, G. Fischer Verlag, Jena.

Pohlmann, R. (1981) *Die Ultraschalltherapie*, Bern.

Repacholli, H.M. (1982) *Ultrasound Characteristics and Biological Action*, National Research Council of Canada, Ottawa.

Roveti, D. (1989) Ultrasound power measurement, *Medical Electronics* **20** (6), 98–106.

Svarcova, J., Trnavsky, K. and Zvarova, J. (1988) The influence of ultrasound, galvanic currents, and shortwave diathermy on pain intensity in patients with osteoarthrosis, *Scand. J. Rheumatol.* **67**, 83–85.

Wells, P.N.T. *Biomedical Ultrasonics*, Academic Press, London.

Wiedau, E. and Röcher, O. (1963) *Ultraschall in der Medizin*, Th. Steinkopff Verlag, Dresden.

Index